Benign Cystic Lesions of the Jaws, their Diagnosis and Treatment

H. C. KILLEY

FDSRCS (Eng.), FDS, HDDRCS (Edin.),
LRCP (Lond.), MRCS (Eng.)

Late Professor of Oral Surgery, London University
Head of Department of Oral Surgery, Eastman Dental Hospital
Hon. Consultant, Eastman Dental Hospital and Westminster
Hospital Teaching Group

L. W. KAY

MDS, FDSRCS (Eng.), LRCP (Lond.), MRCS (Eng.)

Reader in Oral Surgery, London University
Head of the Admissions and Casualty Department, Eastman
  Dental Hospital
Hon. Consultant, Eastman Dental Hospital
Hon. Consultant, Royal London Homeopathic Hospital

G. R. SEWARD

MDS (Lond.), MB, BS (Lond.), FDSRCS (Eng.)

Professor of Oral Surgery, London University,
Head of Department of Oral Surgery, the London Hospital
Medical College,
Hon. Consultant, the London Hospital Group

Benign Cystic Lesions of the Jaws, their Diagnosis and Treatment

H. C. KILLEY

L. W. KAY

G. R. SEWARD

Foreword by
SIR ROBERT BRADLAW CBE, DDSc

Emeritus Professor of Oral Medicine in the University of London
Hon. Professor of Dental Pathology, Royal College of Surgeons of England
Formerly Dean, Institute of Dental Surgery and
Director, Eastman Dental Hospital

THIRD EDITION

CHURCHILL LIVINGSTONE
EDINBURGH LONDON and NEW YORK 1977

CHURCHILL LIVINGSTONE
Medical Division of Longman Group Limited

Distributed in the United States of America by Longman
Inc., 19 West 44th Street, New York, N.Y. 10036 and by
associated companies, branches and representatives
throughout the world.

First Edition 1966
Second Edition . . 1972
Third Edition . . . 1977

ISBN 0 443 01616 X

Printed in Great Britain by
T. & A. Constable Ltd, Edinburgh

Foreword

This admirably succinct account of the diagnosis and treatment of most of the benign cysts of the jaws will be helpful to oral surgeon and dental practitioner alike. Although it is modestly said to be an introduction to the subject rather than a comprehensive study of it, it has the authority and decision that only extensive clinical experience and sound surgical judgment can give. While adequate reference is made to the relevant literature, the basic theme is never obscured by academic controversy regarding aetiological complexities. This is a thoroughly readable book, exemplary in its lucidity and economy of phrase, eminently practical and showing throughout a common-sense approach, which is far from common. I am sure that its readers will find it as informative as I have done.

ROBERT BRADLAW

Preface to the Third Edition

Much important new work has been published since the second edition was produced in 1972, and the text has been thoroughly revised to include some of this material. A new chapter has been introduced on the embryology of the face in relation to cysts of the jaws, and sections have been added on the extrafollicular dentigerous cyst and the calcifying odontogenic cyst. The benign mucosal cyst has been discussed in relation to the differential diagnosis of jaw cysts.

It is hoped that the new edition will continue to prove useful as an introduction to more extensive works on this subject and that it contains an adequate amount of information for undergraduate and postgraduate examinations in dentistry.

H. C. KILLEY
L. W. KAY
G. R. SEWARD

London, 1977

Preface to the First Edition

This monograph has been written for students and practitioners as a guide to the diagnosis and treatment of some of the benign cystic lesions of the jaws. It is not intended as a book on pathology, and only such histopathology as is necessary for a clear understanding of the practical aspects of diagnosis and treatment has been included.

The authors have no wish to enter the controversy concerning the aetiology and classification of these lesions but most of the opposing points of view have, they hope, been fairly stated and discussed. Readers who desire further detail concerning any of these matters are referred to the bibliography of suggested additional reading. It will be seen, therefore, that this book is intended primarily as an introduction and guide to the subject rather than as a comprehensive textbook.

There is some dispute concerning the exact definition of a cyst. A conventional version is that the lesion is an epithelial-lined sac filled with fluid or semi-fluid material, and although all odontogenic and fissural cysts fit this description no allowance is made for such lesions as the solitary bone cyst and Stafne's idiopathic cavity which lack a definitive lining membrane. A more appropriate definition of a cyst is that it is 'an abnormal cavity in hard or soft tissues which contains fluid, semi-fluid or gas and is often encapsulated and lined by epithelium'.

Cysts of the maxilla and mandible are by no means rare and although very small cysts can only be detected radiographically, larger cysts can be diagnosed on careful clinical examination and vigilance by the practitioner will result in their early detection.

Most benign cystic lesions of the jaw tend to increase in size, and as this may eventually lead to serious complications surgical interference is indicated in most instances. There are two main types of operation, enucleation and marsupialisation. Both techniques are comparatively simple and the results are very satisfactory, for recurrence following treatment is exceptional if the operation has been competently performed. In fact, the only benign cystic lesion of the jaws which may occasionally recur is the odontogenic keratocyst and this is probably due to the technical difficulty of removing the very thin cyst lining in its entirety. So far as the convenience of the patient is concerned there is little doubt that enucleation with primary closure is the operative procedure of choice, but marsupialisation is indicated in a certain well-defined group of cases. The relative merits of these two excellent operations are discussed in the appropriate sections of the text.

Undoubtedly the most important aspect of any treatment is the regular post-operative follow-up examination of the lesion, until such time as clinical and radiographic investigations demonstrate that the cyst cavity is obliterated by normal bone.

London, 1966

H. C. KILLEY
L. W. KAY

Acknowledgements

We are indebted to the editor of the *British Dental Journal* for permission to publish the illustrations shown in Figures 5.2, 6.4, 8.2 and 8.3 and to the editor of the *Journal of the International College of Surgeons* for authority to reproduce the illustration numbered Figure 10.1.

We are most grateful to our secretaries, Mrs B. Rayiru and Miss P. A. Hills, BSc, for preparing the manuscript of the first edition and to Miss B. R. Richardson for much painstaking work in preparing the second edition. Mrs B. Rayiru, Mrs G. Clark and Mrs A. McMahon kindly typed the material for the third edition, and the authors wish to thank them most sincerely for their efforts.

We would also like to express our sincere thanks to Dr Victor Goldman, FFA, Consultant Anaesthetist, for taking the photographs appearing in Figures 6.8 to 6.18, and to members of the photographic department of the Eastman Dental Hospital who copied the radiographs.

Mr P. L. James, FDS, MRCS, LRCP, Consultant Oral Surgeon to the London Hospital, was kind enough to allow us to refer to hitherto unpublished material concerning carcinoma arising in an odontogenic cyst and we should like to thank him.

Finally we wish to express our gratitude to Dr W. D. MacLennan, FDS, HDD, LRCP, LRCS, LRFPS, who read the manuscript of the first edition and offered some very helpful suggestions.

HCK
LWK
GRS

Contents

1 Classifications   1

2 Embryology of the face in relation to
  cysts of the jaws   9

3 Signs and symptoms   18

4 Radiology   22

5 Aspiration biopsy   31

6 Treatment   33

7 Odontogenic keratocysts   62

8 Non-keratinizing cysts   75

9 Non-odontogenic cysts   104

10 Bone cysts   119

11 Multiple cysts of the jaws   136

12 Miscellaneous cysts   141

13 Differential diagnosis of cysts of the jaws   151

14 Complications   162

Appendix   169

Index   174

1. Classifications

Classifications are constructed by selecting certain features which are common to a number of conditions and grouping them together on the basis of their shared properties. Depending on the particular features which are selected as the basis for the groupings, a variety of classifications may be constructed. For example, either clinical features, histological appearances, concepts of embryological development or the tissue of origin may form the basis of classification or indeed combinations of these considerations. Ideally, a classification of cysts should be based on their aetiology, but as this is imperfectly understood, the different classifications of cysts of the jaws inevitably reflect advances in knowledge and changing concepts, and different groupings can, by analogy, teach us different things about the conditions concerned. One of the first academic surveys on this subject was conducted by the British Dental Association Committee on Odontomes which published its report in 1914.

The first modern and precise system was devised by Robinson (1945) with the co-operation of other authorities in the field of medicine and dentistry. Antiquated terms were discarded and for classification the cysts were subdivided into two specific groups based on the primal source of the epithelial tissue.

Robinson's classification (1945)

Developmental cysts
(A) From odontogenic tissue
    (1) Periodontal cyst
        (a) Radicular or dental root apex type
        (b) Lateral type
        (c) Residual type
    (2) Dentigerous cyst
    (3) Primordial cyst
(B) From non-dental tissues
    (1) Median cyst (median palatine cyst)
    (2) Incisive canal cyst
    (3) Globulo-maxillary cyst

Robinson's classification was adopted by Thoma and Goldman (1960) with minor modifications, and in this published version the designation follicular cysts is retained and embraces both primordial and dentigerous cysts.

Thoma-Robinson-Bernier classification (1960)

Odontogenic ectodermal epithelial cysts
(A) Follicular cysts
    (1) Primordial cysts
    (2) Dentigerous cysts
        (i) Lateral
        (ii) Central
(B) Periodontal cysts (radicular)
        (i) Apical
        (ii) Lateral
(C) Residual cysts
    (1) Follicular
    (2) Periodontal
(D) Multiple cysts
(E) Multilocular cysts
(F) Polycystoma cysts
(G) Cholesteatoma

Non-odontogenic ectodermal epithelial cysts
(A) Interosseous cysts
    (1) Median
    (2) Intermaxillary
    (3) Nasoalveolar
(B) Nasopalatine cysts
    (1) Incisive canal cysts
    (2) Cyst of papilla palatina

In 1961, Robinson himself expanded his original classification to include cysts of the soft tissues.

Every contemporary authority on cysts has produced a variation of the basic principles in classification formulated by their predecessors. All the later classifications are designed to provide satisfactory groupings of the conditions under consideration without being either too unwieldy or in any way incomplete.

The broad classification offered by Kruger (1964) includes a number of cysts of the soft tissues of the oral cavity and contiguous structures.

Kruger's classification (1964)

(A) Congenital cysts
    (1) Thyroglossal
    (2) Branchiogenic
    (3) Dermoid

(B) Developmental cysts
    (1) Non-dental origin
        (a) Fissural types
            (i) Nasoalveolar
            (ii) Median
            (iii) Incisive canal (nasopalatine)
            (iv) Globulomaxillary
        (b) Retention types
            (i) Mucocele
            (ii) Ranula
    (2) Dental origin
        (a) Periodontal
            (i) Periapical
            (ii) Lateral
            (iii) Residual
        (b) Primordial
        (c) Dentigerous

A classified arrangement of cysts by a British author, Seward (1964), is also noted. The cyst groups are graded in a logical order and range widely in type from cystic neoplasms and bone cysts to the common dental and fissural groups.

Seward's classification (1964)

Cysts with an epithelial lining
(A) From non-odontogenic epithelium
    (1) Maxillary
        (a) Nasopalatine
            (i) Incisive canal cyst
            (ii) Incisive papilla cyst
        (b) Globulomaxillary cyst
        (c) Median palatine cyst
        (d) Nasolabial cyst
    (2) Mandibular
        Median mandibular cyst
(B) From odontogenic epithelium
    (1) Associated with the crown of the tooth
        (a) Cyst of eruption
        (b) Dentigerous cyst
            (i) Pericoronal
            (ii) Lateral
            (iii) Residual
        (c) Extrafollicular dentigerous cyst
    (2) Associated with the root of the tooth

    (a) Inflammatory periodontal or radicular cyst
      (i) Apical
      (ii) Lateral
      (iii) Residual
    (c) Extrafollicular dentigerous cyst
(2) Associated with the root of the tooth
    (a) Inflammatory periodontal or radicular cyst
      (i) Apical
      (ii) Lateral
      (iii) Residual
    (b) Developmental periodontal cyst
(3) Unassociated with a tooth
    (a) Primordial
    (b) Rare entities
      (i) Cyst of interdental papilla
      (ii) Some gingival cysts
(4) Cystic neoplasms (may occur in both solid and cystic form)
    (a) Ameloblastoma
    (b) Adeno-ameloblastoma
    (c) Ameloblastic odontome

Cysts without an epithelial lining
(A) Bone cysts
(B) Stromal cysts in neoplasms

The authors are particularly impressed with the comprehensive classification of Gorlin (1970), and that grouping produced by Lucas (1964) which has the dual advantage of brevity and simplicity. A variety of cysts of the oral tissues and cervicofacial region has been listed by Gorlin, which arbitrarily fall under the headings of intraosseous and soft tissue types, but only those in the former group are relevant to this book. It should be noted that although the word 'fissural' may be inaccurate when applied to some jaw cysts, nevertheless this term is rooted in convention.

Lucas's classification (1964)

Intraosseous cysts
(A) Fisssural cysts
    (1) Median mandibular
    (2) Median palatal
    (3) Nasopalatine
    (4) Globulomaxillary
    (5) Nasolabial
(B) Odontogenic cysts
    (1) Developmental

    (a) Primordial
    (b) Dentigerous
  (2) Inflammatory
  (3) Radicular
(C) Non-epitheliated bone cysts
  (1) Solitary bone cyst
  (2) Aneurysmal bone cyst

Gorlin's classification (1970)
Odontogenic cysts
  (1) Dentigerous cyst
  (2) Eruption cyst
  (3) Gingival cyst of newborn infants
  (4) Lateral periodontal and gingival cysts
  (5) Keratinizing and calcifying odontogenic cyst (cystic keratinizing tumour)
  (6) Radicular (periapical) cyst
  (7) Odontogenic keratocysts
    (a) Primordial cyst
    (b) Multiple keratocyst of jaws, multiple cutaneous nevoid basal cell carcinomas and skeletal anomalies

Non-odontogenic and fissural cysts
  (1) Globulomaxillary (premaxilla-maxillary) cyst
  (2) Nasoalveolar (nasolabial; Klestadt's) cyst
  (3) Nasopalatine (median anterior maxillary) cyst
  (4) Median mandibular cyst
  (5) Anterior lingual cyst
  (6) Dermoid and epidermoid cysts
  (7) Palatal cyst of newborn infants

Cysts of neck, oral floor and salivary glands
  (1) Thyroglossal duct cyst
  (2) Lymphoepithelial ('branchial cleft') cyst
  (3) Oral cysts with gastric or intestinal epithelium
  (4) Salivary gland cyst
  (5) Mucocele and ranula

Pseudocysts of jaws

  (1) Aneurysmal bone cyst
  (2) Static (developmental; latent) bone cyst
  (3) 'Traumatic' (haemorrhagic; solitary) bone cyst

Main (1970) introduced an interesting grouping. He separates cysts of odontogenic epithelium into two groups: primordial cysts, all of which possess the distinctive keratinizing epithelial lining, and dental cysts, under which heading he groups the remaining odontogenic cysts, postulating that they arise in relation to a tooth involved by some preceding pathological process. His remaining group is of cysts arising from non-odontogenic epithelium.

Main's classification (1970)
Primordial cyst
 Replacement
 Envelopmental
 Extraneous
 Collateral

Non-odontogenic
 Median palatal
 Interjacent (globulomaxillary)
 Nasopalatine

Dental
 Coronal
  subfollicular
  inflammatory
 Radicular
 Residual
 Inflammatory collateral

 Replacement primordial cysts are those which are found at the site of a developmentally absent tooth. Envelopmental primordial cysts enclose an entire tooth or at least extend on to the root surface. Extraneous ones arise remote from any teeth and collateral primordial cysts arise in the periodontal membrane of a vital tooth uninvolved by periodontal disease. These would seem to be equivalent to the developmental periodontal cyst of previous authors. In the dental group, the subfollicular coronal cyst covers the anatomical crown of an unerupted tooth, whilst the inflammatory coronal cyst develops around the partly formed crown of a permanent tooth as a result of the intrafollicular spread of periapical inflammation from an overlying deciduous tooth; the radicular and residual cysts are familiar concepts, and the inflammatory collateral forms alongside a partly erupted tooth associated with pericoronitis. A classification of obvious importance is that proposed by the World Health Organization International Reference Centre for the Histological Definition and Classification of Odontogenic Tumours, Jaw Cysts and Allied Lesions.

WHO classification (1971)
Epithelial cysts
(A) Developmental
 (1) Odontogenic

        (a) Primordial cyst (keratocyst)
        (b) Gingival cyst
        (c) Eruption cyst
        (d) Dentigerous (follicular) cyst
    (2) Non-odontogenic
        (a) Nasopalatine duct (incisive canal) cyst
        (b) Globulomaxillary cyst
        (c) Nasolabial (nasoalveolar) cyst
(B) Inflammatory
    Radicular

The preceding classifications are based on the supposed aetiology of each cyst and the elements from which it is presumed to have originated. In some instances the evidence for a contention is convincing, but there is still some controversy concerning the aetiology of, for instance, the solitary bone cyst and the fissural cyst.

Until such problems are resolved no classification of benign cystic lesions of the jaws can rest on a sound scientific basis. In the absence of irrefutable evidence concerning the aetiology and origin of jaw cysts, it is prudent not to be too dogmatic or pedantic in reaching a decision on their classification. The authors have no desire to add to an already long list of excellent classifications, and that chosen for this book is as follows:

(A) *Of odontogenic epithelium*
    (1) Keratocyst
        (a) Primordial cysts
        (b) Extrafollicular dentigerous cysts
    (2) Non-keratinizing
        (a) Cyst of eruption
        (b) Dentigerous
            (i) Pericoronal
            (ii) Lateral
            (iii) Residual
        (c) Radicular
            (i) Apical
            (ii) Lateral
            (iii) Residual
(B) *Of non-odontogenic epithelium*
    (1) Nasopalatine
    (2) Nasoalveolar
(C) *Bone cysts*
    (1) Solitary bone cyst
    (2) Aneurysmal bone cyst

REFERENCES

Gorlin, R. J. (1970) *Thoma's Oral Pathology,* 6th, ed. St Louis: Mosby.
Kruger, G. O. (1964), *Textbook of Oral Surgery,* 2nd. ed. St Louis: Mosby.
Lucas, R. B. (1964) *Pathology of Tumours of the Oral Tissues.* London: Churchill.
Main, D. M. G. (1970) *Brit. J. Oral Surg.,* **8,** 114.
Robinson, H. B. G. (1945) *Am. J. Orthodont.,* **31,** 370.
Seward, G. R. (1964) *Radiology in General Dental Practice.* London: British Dental Association.
Thoma, K. H. & Goldman, H. M. (1960) *Oral Pathology,* 5th ed. St Louis: Mosby.

2. Embryology of the Face in Relation to Cysts of the Jaws

Development of the face

The buccopharyngeal membrane, which marks the site around which the future face will develop, lies initially between the forebrain and the heart in its pericardial sac. Ectomesenchyme from the neural crest flows downwards beneath the epithelium and between the buccopharyngeal membrane and the developing heart. By the fourth week the ectomesenchyme has raised marked ridges in this region to form the mandibular and hyoid arches. Later, further branchial arch ridges are added caudally. Rostral to the buccopharyngeal membrane an accumulation of frontonasal mesenchyme raises a prominence, the so-called frontonasal process. Laterally, first (mandibular) arch mesenchyme flows forwards, subepithelially, to raise further prominences on each side of the buccopharyngeal membrane to form the maxillary processes. As a result, the buccopharyngeal membrane, which at this stage is starting to perforate, lies at the bottom of a broad, shallow pit called the stomatodaeum.

In histological sections the epithelium lateral to the frontonasal mesenchyme is thickened to form the olfactory placodes. Frontonasal mesenchyme medially, above and lateral to the olfactory placodes proliferates to raise a horseshoe-shaped ridge around each placode. Thus during the fifth week the olfactory placodes sink beneath the surface. The medial parts of the ridges are called the medial nasal processes, the lateral parts the lateral nasal processes. At this time the mandibular arches are separated by a median notch, but as the mandibular mesenchyme proliferates medially the notch is smoothed out and a single, complete mandibular arch is established.

During the sixth week the medial nasal processes enlarge considerably, bulging down between the maxillary processes and also growing towards one another. The mesoderm of the two medial nasal processes merges in the midline and smooths out the furrow between them. As a result of their enlargement they overshadow the rest of the frontonasal area. At the same time the maxillary mesoderm increases considerably in volume so that proportionately the distance between the nasal openings is decreased and they appear to come closer together. Further, the maxillary elevations maintain a relationship with the medial nasal processes so that relatively they advance medially below the lateral nasal processes and below the olfactory pits.

As the olfactory placodes sink below the surrounding surface, because of the proliferation of mesenchyme in a horseshoe shape around their borders, they maintain contact with the surface epithelium at their lower edges. The proliferating medial nasal mesenchyme and maxillary mesenchyme therefore cannot intermingle but bulge forwards on either side of a groove at this site and, as the mesenchymal masses enlarge further, the two sides of the groove are pressed together. The two epithelial surfaces adhere to one another and the result is a vertical sheet of epithelium which separates medial nasal and maxillary mesenchyme, and remains attached to the olfactory placode at its upper end. The epithelial sheet is called the nasal fin. Sections show that a small opening forms in the centre of the nasal fin, through which maxillary mesoderm flows. The opening enlarges, either as a result of dilatation by the enlarging mesenchyme, or the retreat of the epithelium towards the new surface level. Epithelial cell rests are an uncommon finding at this site, so that piecemeal destruction as is seen between the palatine processes seems unlikely.

The enlargement of the surrounding parts stretches the remains of the epithelial fin, behind the area of maxillary-medial nasal mesenchymal merger, in a lateral direction. The epithelium at this stage is referred to as the bucconasal membrane, and separates a downwards extension of the olfactory pit from the stomatodaeum. Since this epithelium is not supported by or penetrated by mesoderm, it soon breaks down to establish a communication between the nasal pits and the oral cavity. The openings, one on either side, form the nasal choanae. The tissue below the nasal pits forms the primary palate. Patten (1961) prefers the name 'intermaxillary segment' to 'primary palate' since only the posterior part of the primary palate will contribute to the definitive palate. The middle zone or gnathogingival component will give rise to the premaxillary part of the upper alveolar process and the anterior component will form the medial portion of the upper lip.

The nasolacrimal duct

Where the lateral nasal and maxillary elevations meet there is again a deep grove, the naso-optic furrow or nasolacrimal groove which extends out to the medial corner of the eye. The groove becomes narrowed as a result of mesenchymal growth on either side of it until the epithelial walls are approximated and fuse to form an inwardly directed ridge of epithelium. The ridge subsequently becomes more shallow, either as a result of cell death or cell redistribution. From the region of the upper end of this groove the nasolacrimal duct grows down into the nose (Patten 1961). Whether it arises as a new and separate structure (Politzer 1936) or from the deep surface of the groove remains uncertain. The lateral nasal processes form the alae of the nose.

Development of the palate

During the seventh week shelf-like processes grow out from the sides of the stomatodaeum and in line with the primary palate. Initially the palatal shelves are directed downwards and embrace the tongue on its lateral aspect. As development proceeds the tongue is dislocated from between the palatal shelves which reorientate themselves to grow medially. How this happens is again uncertain. The palatal shelves could actually alter their orientation (Frazer *et al.* 1957, Walker 1961). Once one part of the shelf had achieved a position above the tongue progressive reorientation would displace the tongue downwards. Differential growth of the mandible or oral cavity (Asling *et al.* 1960) and reorientation of the head could exert traction on the tongue, pulling it out from between the palatal processes. Finally Humphrey (1969) suggests that early movements of the mandible which may occur at this age could pull the tongue out from between the palatine processes. In in-vitro experiments it has been noted that removal of the tongue from between the processes results in them assuming the horizontal position immediately (Walker and Frazer 1956, Moriarty *et al.* 1963).

The two epithelium-covered surfaces touch and adhere, and true fusion occurs (Barry 1961). Next the epithelium becomes laminated and less regular in thickness. Holes appear through which the mesoderm on either side merges, and the holes enlarge so that the epithelium breaks up into a series of remnants along the line of contact. These may form epithelial pearls and may be detected in the neonatal period. Because epithelial remnants are not found posteriorly in the soft palate and in the uvula, Bardi (1968) considers that further development and lengthening in this area takes place by merger and backwards displacement of the most posterior point of fusion.

Nasal septum

The posterior nasal openings, or nasal choanae, extend upwards as the surrounding mesoderm increases in bulk and progressively define the nasal septum, the free edge of which faces downwards and backwards. The septum contains frontal and medial nasal mesoderm from between the olfactory pits (Patten 1961), but Baxter (1953) suggests that the extending posterior nasal openings separate off part of the maxillary mesoderm which lies behind the lateral contribution to the septum: Frazer's tectoseptal extension. The nasal septum grows downwards and its free edge fuses with the secondary palate shortly after fusion of the corresponding parts of the palatal processes. The remainder of the free edge forms the posterior border of the nasal septum.

The nasopalatine canals and nasopalatine ducts

Fusion of the palatine processes also takes place with the lateral sides of the triangular-shaped primary palate. This fusion is palatal to the future alveolar process and with the posterior part of Patten's inter-maxillary segment. The last part to unite is the centre of the triradiate line of fusion, and this is the region of the nasopalatine canals.

In certain animals narrow slits are to be found in the palate which open on either side of the nasal septum; these are the nasopalatine canals. In humans there are normally no such openings although very rarely a narrow communication between mouth and nose has been described. Incisive canals are formed in the maxillary bones and these are for the passage of the long spheno-palatine nerves and the terminal parts of the greater palatine arteries. In the region of the developing incisive canals, epithelial cords may be found in the fetus. Some of these are canalized to form tubular structures. Frequently these are blind at both ends, but some open to the surface at one or both ends. These epithelial structures are referred to as naso-palatine ducts (Scott 1955, Abrams *et al.* 1963), but whether they develop as separate and distinct structures or whether they merely represent residues of epithelium from the closure of the triradiate point of union of the primary palate and the palatine processes is not clear.

Development of the tongue

The tongue develops in the floor of the stomatodaeum after the rupture of the buccopharyngeal membrane. During the fifth week lingual swellings arise, one on each side towards the midline of the mandibular arch on its internal aspect. A single medial swelling, the tuberculum impar, is found *caudal* to these swellings, between the first and second arches. The second arch is continuous across the midline, but the third and fourth arches end in a single median eminence, the hypobranchial eminence. Paired swellings arise on the second arch and soon fuse with the front of the hypobranchial eminence to form the copula. At the same time the 'branchial pouch' grooves between the second, third and fourth arches are smoothed out so that distinction between them is lost. On the grounds that the posterior part of the tongue is innervated in the adult by the glossopharyngeal nerve and to a small extent by the vagus, it is suggested that the third and fourth arch tissues flow over and submerge the second arch and its contribution to the tongue.

Anteriorly the lingual swellings from the mandibular arch dominate the scene, enlarging rapidly, fusing with and overgrowing the tuberculum impar. The first arch contribution extends backwards as far as the sulcus terminalis of the definitive tongue and the foramen caecum. Thus the tuberculum impar, which lies immediately anterior to the foramen caecum, plays no part in the formation of the surface of the normal adult tongue.

Tooth development

The first indication of tooth formation is the appearance of condensations of ectomesenchyme with their supportive capillaries under the
epithelium of both upper and lower jaws. These appear first near the
midline then spread progressively backwards in each quadrant. At about
the sixth week the epithelium over these mesodermal condensations
thickens and appears to grow inwards as the primary tooth *band*. The
single band penetrates deeper into the underlying mesenchyme and
divides into two bands; the vestibular band which will degenerate in the
centre to separate the lip from the gum, and the dental lamina which will
produce the tooth germs.

Initially the tooth band in each quadrant is separate, joining subsequently across the midline, and at first the most rapid penetration occurs
at the mesial and distal ends of the band. Epithelial thickening or tooth
buds appear at intervals along the tooth band, and invest the
mesenchymal condensations as the 'cap' stage of the enamel organ with
differentiation of the inner and outer enamel epithelium. With further
differentiation and growth the 'bell' stage is reached, with the appearance
of a fully developed stellate reticulum and the folding of the inner enamel
epithelium to outline the shape of the amelodentinal junction.

As amelogenesis is completed by a particular group of ameloblasts, the
primary enamel cuticle is deposited and the ameloblasts, together with
the remains of the stratum intermedium and external enamel epithelium,
form the reduced enamel epithelium. The stellate reticulum has disappeared from that part by the time amelogenesis is completed.

From the point of union of the external enamel epithelium with the
tooth band, first an extension of the tooth band and then the tooth germ
of the successional tooth develop. The continuous dental lamina breaks
down into a network of epithelial residues and the tooth germs come to
lie deeper in the jaw. Both processes may be related to the increase in
volume of the surrounding tissues.

Where the external and internal enamel epithelia meet at the cervical
margin a double layer of epithelial cells grows down as Hertwig's sheath
to outline the shape of the root. Once the sheath has established the outline of the root and the dentine has been deposited, the sheath becomes
penetrated to form a tenuous network of epithelial cells called the rests of
Malassez.

The merging and fusion of embryonic processes

Peters (1913) and Streeter (1951) emphasized that the grooves
between the so-called processes of the developing face were eliminated by
the elevation of the floor of the groove and not by edge-to-edge contact
and destruction of epithelium. Patten (1961) uses the terms 'fusion',
where epithelium-covered processes cross a gap to unite by their edges

with destruction of the surface epithelia at the point of contact, and 'merging', where a groove or furrow is smoothed out by progressive elevation of its floor. However, he recognizes that in certain situations enlargement of the mesenchymal masses on either side of a groove can occur without the floor being raised up, so that the edges of the groove are pressed together by the bulging eminences on either side. He acknowledges that not only can this occur as a normal mode of development, but also as an abnormal one. A layer of epithelium involved in this way can be eliminated by a subsequent retreat to the surface of the epithelial cells, perhaps as a response to pressure and stretching forces created by rapidly enlarging mesenchyme.

Possible origins of fissural cysts

The possible fissural cysts are:

Maxillary cyst
(a) Nasopalatine
  (i) Incisive canal cyst
  (ii) Incisive papilla cyst
(b) Globulomaxillary cyst
(c) Median alveolar cyst
(d) Median palatine cyst
(e) Nasolabial cyst

Mandibular Cyst
Median mandibular cyst

The existence of nasopalatine cysts is not disputed. These occur in bony cavities which are directly continuous with one or both of the incisive canals and often replace the incisive fossa. The terminal fibres of the long sphenopalatine nerves are normally spread out in the capsule of the cyst. Scott (1955) and Abrams *et al.* (1963) review the origin of these cysts. Epithelial cords, tubes, pearls and microcysts are to be found quite frequently in embryonic material in the incisive canals and cysts forming in the incisive canals or fossae could well develop from this epithelium. These structures are usually referred to as nasopalatine duct remnants, and looked upon as homologous with the nasopalatine canals of other species.

A more superficial cyst occurs in the mucosa behind the incisive papilla. These enlarge and frequently discharge spontaneously, only to enlarge again. They are called cysts of the incisive papilla. Although glandular structures are sometimes seen among the epithelial material in the incisive canals of fetuses, mucous salivary glands are not usually found in the incisive fossa region of normal palates. Occasionally narrow channels may be discovered which are thought to represent persistent tubular nasopalatine duct structures, some of which have been seen to open on to the surface (Abrams *et al.* 1963). If these duct-like structures give rise to the incisive papilla cyst, then they may be looked upon as examples of nasopalatine cysts which lie in the tissues close to the oral cavity.

Whether globulomaxillary cysts exist as entities of developmental origin now seems doubtful. These were popularly ascribed to epithelium at the line of junction between the maxillary and globular process – the latter being the premaxillary process, which is a part of the medial nasal process. Since the nasal fin lies at one stage between maxillary and medial nasal (premaxillary) mesenchyme, the epithelium of the nasal fin could be responsible for globulomaxillary cysts. However, epithelial rests resulting from the breaking of the nasal fin seem to be most uncommon. It is most unlikely that globulomaxillary cysts arise from epithelium trapped between the palatal shelves and the primary palate, for the line of union is behind the alveolar process. This argument is supported by the fact that clefts of the alveolar process are associated with clefts of the lip rather than clefts of the palate.

Most examples of so-called globulomaxillary cysts used as illustrations in publications seem to be apical periodontal (radicular) cysts arising from pulpless lateral incisors, because a cause of pulp necrosis, such as cingulum invagination, or unlined silicate restoration is usually prominent in the radiograph. Seward (1965) has shown how such cysts may well involve the interdental bone between the lateral incisor and canine to produce the pear shape said to be diagnostic of a globulomaxillary cyst.

Sicher (1962) suggested that so-called globulomaxillary cysts were really primordial cysts. If a cyst is found between a vital maxillary lateral incisor and canine it would be an easy matter in these days, unless the cyst were grossly infected, to obtain fluid from the cyst, to estimate the total proteins, to do protein electrophoresis and to obtain a smear from the spun deposit to determine if keratinized cells are present. Further, the operation specimen could be examined to see if the lining had the characteristics of a keratocyst. In this way a diagnosis of primordial cyst could be tested.

Another possible explanation for the occasional cyst which is found between healthy maxillary lateral incisors and canines is that they are residual cysts from the deciduous dentition. If this is so, then such cysts will not have the keratocyst type of lining.

It is now generally accepted that median alveolar cysts do not exist as an entity of developmental origin. Cysts which at one time were described under this name are now recognized as nasopalatine cysts which occupy the lower end of the incisive canal and are projected low down on a periapical film. The mesenchyme of the two median nasal processes merges to smooth out the depression between them early on in development and without any possibility of the entrapment of epithelium between them. Neither the mode of development of the rare median cleft lip nor the cleft of the upper alveolar margin without a cleft lip support the possible occurrence of a median developmental alveolar cyst.

Interestingly, although supernumerary teeth are common in the midline of the upper incisor region and occasionally give rise to dentigerous cysts, primordial cysts are quite uncommon in this region.

Because keratin pearls and microcysts may be found even in the neonate in the midline of the palate and at the line of junction of the palatine shelves, the existence of median palatine cysts has always seemed likely. In fact well-authenticated cases of this entity are virtually unknown and few clinicians now believe in its existence. The explanation would seem to be that the phenomena of microcysts and epithelial pearls at this site in the neonate represents a phase in the destruction of the epithelium rather than its proliferation. The appearance is similar to that seen where cyst lining or palatal epithelium is covered by a soft tissue flap. The epithelium sandwiched between the two layers of connective tissue is broken up and both epithelial pearls and microcysts may be formed before the destruction is complete (Wassmund 1935).

The median mandibular cyst as an entity developing from non-odontogenic epithelium is also discredited (Sicher 1961). Cysts are found in the midline of the mandible which seem to have originated in the midline or from close to the midline. They displace symmetrically the teeth on either side and the lower incisors all respond to vitality tests. Various authors, such as Lucchesi and Topazian (1961) and Blair and Wadsworth (1968) have collected details of such cysts. Both bone cysts and primordial cysts are not uncommon in the lower incisor region and both may account for some cases which have been described. Another type of cyst which could account for other cases is a residual radicular cyst from a deciduous lower central incisor.

Median dermoid cysts are found in the floor of the mouth lingual to the mandible. At an early stage in their development they are found beneath the lingual frenum (Seward 1965). Similar cysts are found in the midline of the tongue and it is likely that they arise from epithelium trapped between the two lingual swellings which enlarge backwards from the mandibular arch to form the anterior two-thirds of the tongue. The median mandibular cysts do not seem to be similar histologically to these sublingual dermoids and do not seem to be related.

The nasolabial cyst is found beneath the ala of the nose and the adjacent part of the upper lip. Because no subperiosteal new bone is formed over its surface it must develop extraperiosteally (Seward 1962). Even so it causes a saucer-shaped depression in the adjacent alveolar process and alters the shape of the anterior bony aperture of the nose. It develops therefore at the lower end of the line of junction of the maxillary and lateral nasal elevations. As was noted earlier the naso-optic furrow which lies between these two processes forms an inwardly directed ridge of epithelium, and there would seem to be an opportunity for sequestration of the inner part of this ridge and hence for the development of a nasolabial cyst.

The development of odontogenic cysts is more conveniently dealt with later and will be found in the appropriate chapters.

REFERENCES
Abrams, A. M., Howell, F. V. & Bullock, W. K. (1963) *Oral Surg.,* **16,** 306.
Asling, C. W., Nelson, M. M. Dougherty, H. L., Wright, H. V. & Evans, H. M. (1960), *Surg. Gynec. Obstet.,* **111,** 19.
Bardi, A. R. (1968) *J. Oral Surg.,* **26,** 41.
Barry, A. (1961) Development of the branchial regions of the human embryo; in *Congenital Anomalies of the Face and Associated Structures,* ed. S. Pruzansky. Illinois: Thomas.
Baxter, J. S. (1953) *Frazer's Manual of Embryology,* 3rd ed. London: Baillière.
Blair, A. E. & Wadsworth, W. (1968) *J. Oral Surg.,* **26,** 735.
Brandt, W. & Roper-Hall, H. T. (1941) *Brit. Dent. J.,* **70,** 213.
Frazer, C. F., Walker, B. E. & Trasler, D. T. (1957) *Pediatrics,* **19,** 782.
Humphrey, T. (1969), *Amer. J. Anat.,* **25,** 317.
Lucchesi, F. J. & Topazian, D. S. (1961) *J. Oral Surg.,* 19, 336.
Moriarty, T. M., Weinstein, S. & Gibson R. D. (1963) *J. Embryol. Exp. Morph.,* **11,** 605.
Patten, B. M. (1961) Normal development of the facial region; in *Congenital Anomalies of the Face and Associated Structures,* ed. S. Pruzansky. Illinois: Thomas.
Peters, K. (1913) *Atlas der Entwicklung der Nase und des Gaumens beim Menschen.* Jena: Gustav Fisher.
Politzer, G. (1936) *Anat.,* **97,** 557.
Roper-Hall, H. T. (1938) *Brit. Dent. J.,* **65,** 405.
Scott, J. H. (1955) *Brit. Dent. J.,* **98,** 109.
Seward, G. R. (1962) *Dent. Pract.,* **12,** 154.
Seward, G. R. (1965) *Brit. J. Oral Surg.,* **3,** 36.
Sicher, H. (1962) *Oral Surg.,* **15,** 1264.
Streeter, G. L. (1951) *Developmental horizons in human embryology age groups 11 to 23.* Carnegie Contrib. to Emb. Reprint Vol. 2.
Walker, B. E. & Frazer, F. C. (1956) *J. Embryol. Exp. Morph.,* **4,** 176.
Walker, F. C. (1961) Experimental induction of cleft palate; in *Congenital Anomalies of the Face and Associated Structures,* ed. S. Pruzansky. Illinois: Thomas.
Wassmund, M. (1935) *Lehrbuch der praktischen Chirurgie des Mundes und der Kiefer,* Band 1. Liepzig: Meusser.

3. Signs and Symptoms

Physical signs

The physical signs of a cyst in the jaws must, of course, depend upon the size of the cyst. If the cyst is small and has not produced expansion of the jaw, there will be no demonstrable signs to indicate its presence. Usually such lesions are discovered during a routine radiological examination. In the case of a very small apical periodontal cyst the presence of a dead tooth or residual root may suggest the possibility of an underlying pathological condition, but in fact only a minimal percentage of dead teeth have periapical cysts.

As the cyst becomes larger, expansion of the alveolar bone occurs. Frequently, only the labial or buccal aspect of the lower jaw is affected in the case of an odontogenic cyst, and a swelling of the lingual plate alone or involvement of both inner and outer bony walls may be indicative of a different type of lesion. Although in common usage, the term 'expansion' is not a strictly accurate interpretation of the change which takes place when a growing cyst causes a local discernible distension or bulging of the external bony surface. As a cyst increases in size the periosteum is stimulated to form a layer of new bone, and it is this subperiosteal deposition which alters the outline of the affected portion of the jaw and produces a curved enlargement. At an early stage the lateral expansion presents a smooth, hard, painless prominence, but as cyst growth proceeds the bone covering the centre of the convexity becomes thin and can be depressed with pressure in a manner similar to indenting the surface of a table-tennis ball. With further expansion, the fragile outer shell of bone becomes fragmented; the sensation imparted and sound produced on palpation over the area have been described as 'egg-shell crackling'. Later, these small pieces of bone diappear and are not replaced by a layer of new bone. Now the cyst lining lies immediately beneath the mucosa and fluctuation can be elicited (Fig. 3.1). At this stage if the finger is run along the buccal sulcus the fluctuant area is found to be bounded by a firm, resistant bony shelf which slopes gradually into the normal contour of the jaw. Greater distension of the wall of the cyst sac leads to eventual discharge of fluid into the mouth, a situation which is frequently followed by secondary infection and the formation of a soft tissue abscess. This sequence of events is commonly observed with progressive enlargement of periodontal and dentigerous cysts. Because odontogenic keratocysts tend to develop in parts of the jaws where ex-

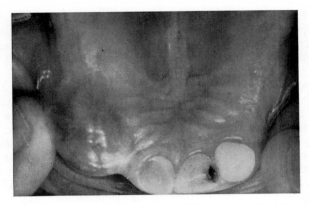

Fig. 3.1 The physical sign of fluctuation could be elicited on palpating this swelling in the /3 region which was due to a residual periodontal cyst.

pansion is less evident and because they may not cause symptoms until a late stage their enlargement may be overlooked. Solitary bone cysts also remain symptomless for long periods and likewise only cause expansion of the jaws at a late stage of their development. Fissural cysts are usually small but occasionally a nasopalatine cyst may attain a considerable size and resemble the more common periodontal cyst in clinical features.

From the point of view of site, periodontal and dentigerous cysts may occur anywhere in the mouth, but in the former case upper teeth are predominantly affected, especially the lateral incisor, whilst the latter are most frequently associated with impacted or displaced canines, premolars and lower third molars. Fissural cysts are, of course, confined to the upper jaw, and solitary bone cysts virtually to the mandible. Stafne's idiopathic bone cavities are habitually located beneath the mandibular canal at the lower border of the mandible, and odontogenic keratocysts are often seen in the lower third molar area and extend into the ramus.

Benign cysts rarely cause loosening of adjacent teeth until the cyst is very large. The clinical absence of one or more teeth from the normal series in an otherwise complete dentition without a history of preceding extraction may imply the presence of a developing dentigerous cyst. A single missing tooth may also invite suspicion of the existence of an odontogenic keratocyst of the primordial type.

Although large mandibular cysts invariably involve the neurovascular bundle and even deflect this structure into an abnormal position, it is unusual to find anaesthesia of the mental distribution of the nerve. If an acute infection of a cyst should occur due to the existence of a communication between the cyst and the oral cavity, then a sudden increase in pressure from pus accumulating in the sac will cause a neurapraxia of the nerve and the immediate onset of labial anaesthesia. When tension is

B

relieved by spontaneous discharge of pus or surgical drainage of the infected cyst, sensation will return to normal. In contrast an uninfected benign cyst grows so slowly and exerts such slight pressure on the neurovascular bundle over a long period of time that anaesthesia does not result.

The teeth adjoining an odontogenic keratocyst, a fissural cyst or a solitary bone cyst will have vital pulps unless there is coincidental disease of these teeth. Apical periodontal cysts are associated with a pulpless tooth, but in the case of lateral periodontal cysts the involved tooth is often vital. Surprisingly, erupted teeth related to a large cyst may remain vital even though the supporting bone has largely been lost. With infected cysts there may be temporary absence of a vital response in adjacent teeth due to pressure interference with sensory transmission in the pulp.

The absence of a tooth together with a cystic swelling may suggest the presence of a dentigerous cyst.

Occasionally, percussion of the teeth overlying a solitary bone cyst produces a 'dull' or 'hollow' sound in contrast to the high-pitched note obtained on tapping normal teeth on the opposite side of the jaw.

If the cyst has discharged into the mouth a sinus may be present and on probing this a bony cavity is found. A thin, watery fluid may be expressed from such a sinus when the expanded wall of the cyst is pressed. The fluid can be examined for cholesterol crystals. A gush of fluid released by the extraction of a tooth may be the first indication of the presence of a cyst. If a tooth is extracted from over a large cyst a circular opening will remain at the site of the socket and will not heal. In the maxilla such an opening may be mistaken for an antro-oral fistula. The decompression will stimulate the cyst to fill in. Evidence of suppuration within a cyst will be provided by the cardinal signs of infection, i.e. increased swelling, tenderness, reddening and pain. However, because of the large volume of pus which may be present the toxaemia will be out of proportion to what would be expected from an apical abscess.

In the edentulous patient a previously comfortable, well-fitting denture may become dislodged by an expanding cyst, and at the point where the plate cuts into the growing lesion a denture granuloma may develop. Where a denture has been worn for some years inspection of the fitting surface may disclose a depression as evidence that the cyst was already present when the denture was constructed.

The cystic nature of a lump may often be demonstrated by applying firm interrupted pressure with a finger of one hand over the suspected lesion in the buccal sulcus and detecting the transmitted impulse with another finger placed on the opposite side of the lesion. As the sensation of fluctuance is conveyed via the cystic fluid, the test will be negative if the cyst is multilocular. When fluctuation is elicited due to resorption of the buccal surface of the alveolus as the cyst bulges outwards, it may be possible to identify the bluish colour of the cyst beneath the oral mucous membrane.

A large anterior maxillary cyst may extend under the nasal floor or cause distortion of the nostril. Involvement of the antrum by an infected cyst may produce signs of maxillary sinusitis.

Large cysts in the maxilla frequently displace the roots of the cheek teeth buccally so that the crowns are inclined palatally. In either jaw a cyst enlarging between two teeth will cause their roots to diverge and their crowns to converge. Later the adjacent teeth (usually on one side only) will tilt over as well, like a row of packing cases which have fallen sideways.

Symptoms

Usually if the cyst is small, the patient is symptomless. Often the first symptom a patient experiences is pain and swelling when the cyst becomes infected. Sometimes a patient notices a lump in the sulcus, and occasionally, in the case of a dentigerous cyst, the patient may seek advice concerning a tooth missing from the dentition.

If the cyst is large the patient may first request treatment when a pathological fracture has occurred in the weakened jaw. It is surprising how few symptoms this may cause – sometimes only a click, followed by mild discomfort and a progressive but slight disturbance to the occlusion.

If the cyst has discharged into the mouth and becomes secondarily infected, the patient may express concern about a nasty taste. Patients with fissural cysts often complain of a salty taste when a sinus is present. Occasionally, an infected cyst is mistaken for a common dental abscess and a tooth is extracted. The discharge of pus from the socket will prevent healing and the patient may present complaining of a painful dry socket. As this heals a permanent wide sinus is left into the cyst cavity and infection will follow, perhaps with the accumulation of food debris therein. Edentulous patients may have found that their denture has become gradually displaced or is cutting into the gum and causing pain or a denture ulcer.

Any cyst may displace adjoining teeth, and the patient may have become aware of an irregularity of the dentition. A non-vital tooth associated with a periapical cyst may become discoloured and/or slightly loose – and this may form the patient's complaint.

4. Radiology

The classic radiological appearance of a common odontogenic cyst in the jaws is that of a well-defined, round or oval area of radiolucency, circumscribed by a sharp radio-opaque margin. However, there are many variations to this standard pattern which depend not only upon cyst type but are related to location and the degree of bone destruction and expansion. There are, too, radiolucencies suggestive of a cyst formation which are caused by other pathological entities and these represent potential pitfalls for the unwary. For example, the monocular rarefaction produced by a central benign neoplasm may be misdiagnosed as a cystic cavity, and a multicystic formation can be simulated by giant-cell lesions, haemangiomata and adamantinomata. Indeed the only reason for describing this particular appearance with confidence as representing a cyst is because cysts of the jaws are so common and, by comparison, the solid soft tissue lesions are uncommon.

Confusion may also arise as a result of the cyst-like contour of normal anatomical structures. For instance the incisive fossa may be misinterpreted as a developmental cyst, and the shadow of the mental foramen superimposed over the apex of a premolar tooth may be mistaken for a small periodontal cyst. Another anatomical landmark which has to be differentiated from a cystic condition is the maxillary sinus.

In diagnostic radiology for cysts of the jaws a minimum of two films should be taken at right angles to each other. Usually with large cysts in either jaw extraoral radiography is an essential supplement to conventional intraoral views.

Intraoral radiography

The requisite intraoral projections are periapical films, a standard occlusal view and a lateral or topographical occlusal view.

Periapical films

These should provide a distinct and accurate image of the cystic area visualized, but because of the small size of standard films only a portion of a large cyst cavity may be shown. It is important to take periapical radiographs near the ends of large cysts so that their extremities are well defined. When the cyst reduces the thickness of the cortex a reduction in the exposure may be appropriate and produce a more informative radiograph.

Standard occlusal view
In the upper jaw this type of radiograph will reveal the amount of palatal bone destruction caused by a cystic process and disclose any alteration to the bony contour of the maxilla from cyst expansion outwards. An occlusal view of the long axis of the mandible will reveal characteristic 'distension' of the inner or outer cortical plates.

Topographical occlusal view
This ancillary occlusal view is useful in differentiating a cystic condition from the antral shadow, and it also eliminates superimposition of the zygomatic bone over the apices of a molar which might have been responsible for the pathological change.

Extraoral radiography

Extraoral radiography should demonstrate the full extent of the abnormality and provide an accurate reproduction of the normal marginal bone encompassing the lesion.

Oblique lateral views
An image of the body of the mandible can be obtained by segmental examination from the symphyseal region to the angle. Specifically this profile projection is valuable in defining a cyst cavity encroaching upon or perforating the lower border, for assessing the degree of involvement of the ramus and for demonstrating displacement of the inferior dental canal and migration of teeth. The greater length of jaw covered by these films integrates the separate images in periapical films when a larger cyst is investigated. They do not replace the periapical films, as they lack the image definitions of the latter.

Posterior-anterior projection
This radiograph provides a comprehensive survey of the mandible – symphysis, body and rami – and will disclose lateral and medial expansion of the ramus.

Lateral sinuses view
An excellent projection for (1) localizing a high, unerupted tooth associated with a large maxillary dentigerous cyst, (2) determining the upper margin of a large odontogenic cyst invading the antrum, and (3) delineating the limits of a mucous cyst of the maxillary sinus.

Occipitomental view
This is complementary to the above in the study of cysts occupying a part or the whole of the antral space. Because of the tilt of the head, anterior cysts are well seen and their size relative to the antrum accentuated. Cysts originating posteriorly may be concealed until they are of considerable size. A well-penetrated PA jaws view may be more valuable for a posterior cyst.

Rotational tomography

Both the orthopantomogram and the Panelipse produce markedly better radiographs and involve a more simple technique than the earlier machines. So much better are these films, and because the whole of the affected jaw is displayed, they replace to a considerable degree the oblique lateral radiograph. The only consideration is both the cost of the machine and the higher cost of the films. Because the technique is a tomographic one and the image represents a layer of tissue the less complex mandible is more easily displayed and interpreted than the maxilla. Where the plane of cut crosses a depression in the surface of the bone, as in the region of the canine fossa in the maxilla, an appearance closely resembling a cyst may be produced. Artifacts of this nature must be borne in mind when interpreting these films.

Tomography has been employed in the examination of cysts of the jaws, but its application in this field is very restricted in view of the excellent information afforded by routine views. Nevertheless, it would seem apposite to use this method when greater clarity is required in the radiological investigation of cystic destruction in the region of the condylar and coronoid processes, and rotational tomography is not to hand. It could also be employed to define the outline of an expanded maxilla.

Stereoscopy

Stereoscopy is a technique for obtaining perspective or depth in the radiographic mental image. The principle has been applied to the localization of unerupted teeth, and stereoscopic studies might be used to determine the exact position of a bony cavity or to overcome limitations in radiographic interpretation when involvement of tooth apices by a cyst is queried. For routine purposes stereoscopic projections should not be used if single plane films will suffice.

Interpretation

In cyst interpretation it is necessary to remember some simple basic facts:

1. Small cysts in cancellous bone are round, but as they become larger their circular shape tends to be lost due to the differing degrees of peripheral resistance offered to their expansion. Contact with mandibular cortical plates retards the rate of growth laterally and medially, and, therefore, increase in size tends to take place along the longitudinal axis at the expense of the less solid cancellous tissue which provides a path of reduced resistance. Consequently, in the mandible a cyst may extend along the whole length of the jaw and assume an elongated sausage shape with minimal discernible external deformity.

When expansion of the cortex does occur in the mandible, there is a tendency for it to be more pronounced on the labial or buccal aspects. The exception to this trend is encountered in the third molar area where lingual precedes lateral expansion, presumably because of the thickness of buccal plate at that site and the lingual position of the wisdom tooth or its developing tooth germ.

2. In an occlusal radiograph of a periodontal cystic area in which erupted teeth have been tilted, the tooth which is not out of line is the cause of the cyst. The radiographic images of such deflected teeth are foreshortened, and a modification of the angle of projection in periapical radiography may be appropriate. Standing teeth may also be rotated by an expanding cyst, and pressure exerted by a cystic lesion on a developing root may result in dilaceration of the corresponding subsequently calcified portion.

3. When either or both mandibular cortical plates are perforated as a result of continuing bony destruction by a cyst, the hole through the bone is evidenced by a well-demarcated, dark shadow which is superimposed upon the fainter image of the remainder of the cystic space in which a residual bone structure is preserved. Where the images of perforations of both cortical plates partly overlap, a complex image is produced suggestive of a multilocular cavity.

4. The presence of a large cyst in the mandible may cause downwards and lateral displacement of the dark band of the inferior dental canal and a discontinuity in one or both cortical lines which outline this canal, so that at operation the neurovascular contents would be within the fibrous capsule of the cyst. After the lining has been dissected out they will be found to be exposed along the floor of the cavity.

5. Maxillary cysts discovered radiologically are often large in size although there may be no clinically detectable expansion.

6. The inclusion of an unerupted tooth in an area of radiolucency does not necessarily imply a dentigerous cyst formation (Fig. 4.1). The tooth may have been intimately associated with a neoplasm or another type of cyst, the enlargement of which has enclosed the tooth at an early stage or moved it so that it lies somewhere along the periphery of the lesion and has become partially enveloped. A cyst will displace a tooth much more readily in a young person's jaw than in that of an adult individual.

7. When an unerupted tooth has a large follicular space around its crown the question of dentigerous cyst formation arises. There is no accepted normal limit for follicle size. The follicular space may increase to twice the width considered normal during development of the crown at the time when the tooth is about to erupt. A follicle which is three times the normal width should be viewed with suspicion. In doubtful cases radiographs should be repeated at intervals over a suitable period of time to determine if there has been an increase in the dimensions of the space. An impacted tooth with a widened follicle should be removed. An unimpacted tooth with a widened follicular space which fails to erupt normally should be explored and the follicular tissues submitted for biopsy.

8. Multilocularity is often fictitious, being a projection effect of the elevations or ridges in the cyst walls which are consequent upon differential bone resorption. Scalloping or lobulation along the margin of the ac-

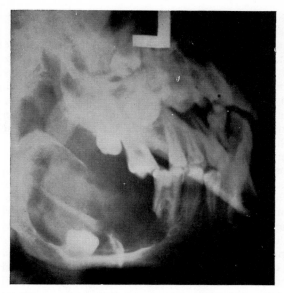

Fig. 4.1 Lateral oblique radiograph of a monocystic lesion causing resorption of the distal root of 6/. This is an adamantinoma but it could be confused with a dentigerous cyst.

tual area of cavitation is also due to uneven loss of bone. Apparent cyst loculation in the ramus may be due to superimposition upon the radiolucency of bony ridges along which slips of the masseter muscle are attached, or to perforations of the cortex.

9. As a cyst heals the circumferential white line fades, and gradually the cavity is eliminated by cancellous bone deposition from the periphery inwards. Initially the bone is deposited as trabeculae which radiate inwards from the internal surface of the bony cavity. Alveolar bone regenerates around the apices of vital teeth over which the cyst has extended. Eventually the replacement osseous tissue assumes the normal radiological pattern and density of the surrounding bone. However, it is not unusual in the case of a nasopalatine cyst for the radiolucent defect to persist or to undergo incomplete bony repair, perhaps due to the absence or partial destruction of periosteum. Following treatment of a cyst which has occupied the maxillary sinus and displaced or eroded the cavity walls, the antral space assumes its former shape and its boundaries reform.

10. In the young adult it is unusual for a palatal cyst to cross the midline because of the restraining influence of the median suture. About the fifth decade the limiting suture closes, but a longstanding cyst in an older patient may cross the midline even before this date.

To assist in the differential diagnosis between cyst and maxillary sinus, it may be necessary to use intraoral periapical films, occlusal views and the occipitomental projection. There are certain points of distinction which help to make a decision:

1. The antrum has some bony pattern due to overlying cancellous bone and the anatomical markings of the neurovascular canals cross the shadow of the space, and appear as dark lines running mainly in an antero-posterior direction. In contrast the cyst cavity is a structureless dark area, and if the capsular vessels are visible it is only for a short distance or end on.

2. The maxillary sinuses are frequently symmetrical, and although an apparent discrepancy in configuration may represent a normal anatomical variation it may also signify the presence of a pathological condition such as a cyst.

3. When a cyst fills the greater part of the antral cavity, a periapical film of the tuberosity region may show two adjacent and parallel white lines, the inner of which defines the margin of a cyst, and the outer the sharply etched boundary of the sinus. In a lateral sinuses view, a similar double outline is of less significance and probably depicts a superimposition of the image of one antrum upon the other.

4. An important diagnostic landmark is reputed to to be the Y-shaped line of Ennis. The forking limbs of the Y formation delineate the anterior wall of the sinus swinging away from the lateral wall of the nose. A horizontal continuation posteriorly of the latter (or more precisely the line of junction of the lateral wall and the nasal floor) is represented by the long leg of the letter Y. In the crotch of the Y is cancellous bone supporting the first premolar, canine and incisors. Effacement or modification of the typical pattern may follow cystic development and growth in the area. However, if a cyst becomes large enough to displace the maxillary sinus from this part of the alveolar process and replace it in relation to the inferior meatus, then a new Y-shaped configuration will be formed by the cyst and the floor of the nose. In such cases asymmetry between the right and left sides in the antero-posterior position of the Y may draw attention to the cyst.

5. Apart from the possibility of undulations of the antral floor between the teeth, bony septa may exist which partition the cavity into loculi or even produce a single division of the space into two distinct compartments forming a double curve and resembling the letter W above the apices of the molar teeth (McCall and Wald 1957). It is essential to distinguish normal loculation from the globular shadows of dental cysts, and also to interpret correctly the dark areas caused by antral recesses or pouches.

6. An occlusal view demonstrates that the anterolateral wall of the antrum has a concave outline, but a cyst expanding the bone in this region converts this linear concavity into a thin, convex, bow-shaped border.

7. Although in an intraoral film a maxillary cyst produces an area of radiolucency, if the fluid-filled sac breaches the floor of the sinus and protrudes into the cavity it will appear on an occipitomental film as a

rounded uniform opacity. The relative increase in density is attributable to the radiological contrast effect of the fluid content in a normally translucent air space. A projection taken with the patient's head tilted will demonstrate that the convex superior border of the cyst maintains an identical relationship to the sinus walls as that shown on the standard view taken in a straight position. In contradistinction, free fluid in the antrum (such as pus) assumes a new horizontal level and a mucous cyst of the maxillary sinus will flop sideways and change shape. Compared with a mucous cyst the thin layer of expanded bone over a cyst arising from within the alveolar process will produce a more distinct and radio-opaque margin. As the cyst expands and replaces the air, the radiolucent image of the sinus cavity contracts in size and eventually the whole air space is obliterated by a homogeneous opaque shadow.

8. A cyst may deform, evaginate, thin or erode a lateral wall of the antrum, and sometimes appears to cross both lateral and medial walls and even protrude into the nasal fossa. Where a cyst expands towards the lateral side and floor of the inferior meatus it will eventually bulge towards the nasal cavity. The normal lateral convexity in an antero-posterior direction of the wall of the inferior meatus will be reversed. While a cyst may cross the midline in the palatal bone and bulge into both nasal fossae, the cartilaginous nasal septum persists and permanently indents the upper surface.

9. The roots of healthy teeth projecting into the normal antral cavity have an intact lamina dura, but in periodontal cyst formation the lamina dura of the causative tooth is absent apical to the point of attachment. The clear-cut cancellous bone margin which circumscribes the pathological area of radiolucency merges with the remaining lamina dura. Usually the dead tooth will be carious, and if this is not evident radiographically in the case of a lateral incisor a dens invaginatus may be present.

10. In a radiograph the apices of adjacent teeth may be overlapped by the clearly defined dark area of an odontogenic cyst and partly denuded of lamina dura. Sometimes the discontinuity of the lamina dura may be more apparent than real. Sometimes the apices of the teeth overshadowed by a cyst undergo resorption due to a longstanding pressure effect. The outline of the resorption is usually continuous with the cyst margin.

11. The margins of the maxillary sinus are thin, discrete and irregular in an intraoral view, but the border of a cyst is curved under pressure from its contents. Rarely a cyst may show calcification in its walls.

12. In his monograph, Sonesson (1950) claimed that 80 per cent of the cases in his series of cysts had no visible cortical margin. Pertinent to this statement, Seward (1964) has pointed out that, with certain provisos, if a cavity in the maxilla is separated from the cancellous bone by a white cortical line it is likely to be the sinus, but if there is no white line it is probably a cyst.

13. According to Seward, a differentiating characteristic is that the

maxillary sinus expands into the alveolar process from above, whereas the cyst originates from within the process. A cystic cavity having a short antero-posterior diameter will usually have its inferior border lower in the ridge than an intruding sinus, and its upper boundary will be detectable in suitable films.

14. A mucosal cyst of the antrum must be distinguished from an odontogenic cyst. The former is usually dome-shaped, uniformly radio-opaque and well defined, but bereft of a white marginal line. It does not displace the walls of the antrum as may an odontogenic cyst. The view of Bret-Day (1960) is that a dental cyst expanding the antral floor would give a similar appearance to a secretory cyst, but the angle formed by the antral floor and cyst wall would be less acute.

Other radiological diagnostic techniques

If it is still difficult to make a confident diagnosis, aspiration and the injection of a contrast medium are alternative technical aids.

The introduction of a radio-opaque medium into a cystic lesion is a rarely used investigation for distinguishing cyst from sinus. The injection of a water-soluble contrast solution by a wide-bore needle into the cavity to be explored is preceded by withdrawal of any fluid content. Both during the withdrawal of the fluid and during the subsequent injection it is important to have a second needle entering the cyst cavity to prevent adverse changes in pressure within the cyst. Toller's double-lumen needle (Toller 1970) is a satisfactory way of avoiding a negative pressure during aspiration and painful positive pressure during the injection. The dense shadow outlining the cyst space can be shown by standard radiographs. Insufficient filling of the cavity could lead to incorrect interpretation, but on the other hand a small amount of opaque medium can be used to define the dimensions of a large cyst by moving the head so that any fluid level is parallel with the film when the radiograph is taken.

Injections should not be given with great force, for if the separation between the lesion and the sinus is merely a thin cyst capsule, the soft tissue partition may rupture. Care should also be taken to avoid overflow into the soft tissues, which distorts the picture by superimposing opacities. The absorption and elimination of Hypaque is excellent, but it is contraindicated in patients with severe renal disease and hepatic disorders, and it may cause a hypersensitivity reaction in patients with an allergic diathesis.

After the essential radiographs have been taken, it may be advisable to remove the contrast material by aspiration or other methods. If a large opening into the cavity exists, moving the patient's head so that the outlined space is no longer in a dependent position will permit the fluid to drain out. Water-soluble medium will disperse itself.

Other indications for radio-opaque fluid in the investigation of cysts are (1) to demonstrate the relationship of a nasolabial cyst to the surface of the maxilla and to the margins of the anterior nasal aperture, and (2) to produce sialographic evidence that a Stafne's cavity may contain a lobule of the submandibular salivary gland.

Contrast medium can also be utilized after treatment of the cyst – to follow the progress of regression of a marsupialized cavity. The cavity can be packed with a bismuth-iodoform paste impregnated pack for the purpose of radiography. With later follow-ups at six-monthly intervals, cotton wool soaked in Lipiodol can be substituted for this purpose.

REFERENCES

Bret-Day, R. C. (1960) *Brit. dent. J.*, **109**, 268.
McCall, J. O. & Wald, S. S. (1957) *Clinical Dental Roentgenography*, 4th ed. Philadelphia: Saunders.
Seward, G. R. (1964) *Radiology in General Dental Practice*. London: British Dental Association.
Sonesson, A. (1950) *Acta Radio.* Suppl. 81.
Toller, P. A. (1970) *Brit. dent. J.*, **128**, 317.

5. Aspiration

Aspiration of a suspected cyst is a valuable diagnostic aid, especially when doubt still exists about the nature of the lesion after careful clinical and radiological examination. This investigation is also helpful in distinguishing between a maxillary cyst and the maxillary sinus (Fig. 5.1). A wide-bore needle should be inserted into the suspected cystic lesion under local analgesia and the cavity then aspirated. A provisional diagnosis of benign cyst will be confirmed if the aspirate withdrawn is a light, straw-coloured fluid containing cholesterol crystals. The presence of cholesterol crystals is easily demonstrated by running some of the aspirated fluid on to a dry swab, for the crystals can be identified by their characteristic shimmering effect when viewed in a strong light. On microscopical examination the distinctive shape of a cholesterol crystal is rectangular with one corner missing.

If the needle has been inserted into the maxillary sinus, aspiration of air will occur, and the diagnosis can be verified by injecting into the space about 20 ml of sterile distilled water which will run out through the nasal ostium and pass down the nostril.

The cavity of the maxillary sinus may be occupied by a large, mucous cyst which radiographically will be seen to have a convex surface (Fig. 5.2). On aspiration, pale, straw-coloured fluid containing perhaps a few cholesterol crystals will be obtained. In some cases the fluid will clot, unlike the fluid from a radicular or dentigerous cyst. This condition is com-

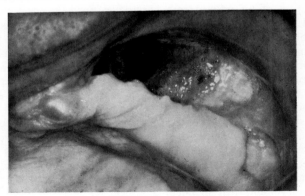

Fig. 5.1 This is a maxillary sinus which was marsupialized in the mistaken belief that it was an odontogenic cyst. The patient was referred for closure of the defect.

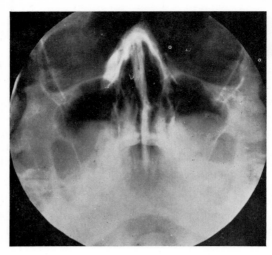

Fig. 5.2 An occipitomental projection which reveals bilateral opaque shadows with convex upper margins occupying part of the antra. These represent mucous cysts of the maxillary sinus.

paratively rare, and confusion between a mucous cyst of the antrum and a benign odontogenic cyst seldom arises.

If aspiration is attempted on a solid lesion, not only is nothing aspirated, but it is impossible to withdraw the plunger of the syringe. The ability to aspirate a syringe full of blood without difficulty should lead the operator to suspect either a central cavernous haemangioma or an aneurysmal bone cyst. In the case of a solitary bone cyst the characteristic aspirate is a golden-yellow fluid which clots on standing. The supernatant fluid over the clot or anticoagulated fluid should be tested for bilirubin, and a substantial amount is usually present.

Aspiration of an odontogenic keratocyst produces pale yellow, inspissated material which appears to be pus, but is in fact liquid containing masses of desquamated keratinized cells. The absence of an offensive odour, together with the lack of confirmation of secondary infection in the history of the lesion, will assist in making the correct diagnosis.

Infected cysts contain pus and normal cyst fluid. After longstanding infection the cyst may be filled with a thick, semi-solid, yellow or brown mass, and cholesterol crystals which cannot be aspirated.

Analysis of aspirated cyst fluid by paper electrophoresis appears to be of diagnostic value, serving to differentiate the keratocyst from other odontogenic cyst types. It also has the ancillary advantage of assisting the surgeon in his treatment plan, since the surgical approach in the case of a keratocyst may have to be more radical. Details of the differentials in protein level and their significance appear on page 68. A smear of the cyst fluid also can be prepared and stained to demonstrate the typical keratinized cells.

6. Treatment

There are several excellent reasons why benign cysts need treatment. Firstly, these cysts increase in size and eventually become infected. Their presence in the jaw constitutes an area of weakness which, particularly in the case of the mandible, may result in a pathological fracture. It is also impossible to be absolutely certain of the nature of a lesion, even if it has been demonstrated to be cystic, until it has been explored surgically and a specimen of tissue has been examined histologically. For example, both ameloblastomas and mucoepidermoid salivary carcinomas are likely to be slow-growing and can produce cystic swellings which mimic benign cysts. Finally, important neighbouring structures may be involved or encroached upon. For instance, adjacent erupted or unerupted teeth may be displaced, tilted, resorbed or their bony support reduced. Moreover, the maxillary sinus or inferior meatus of the nose may be encroached upon, resulting in nasal obstruction, recurrent sinusitis, or even epiphora if the nasolacrimal duct is occluded.

However, benign cysts are often slow-growing and it may be reasonable merely to keep under regular review a small cyst in an elderly or infirm patient. Under certain conditions, which will be mentioned in later chapters, some cysts regress and disappear. Generally speaking, observation in expectation of such a happening is very rarely advisable, but the possibility can be kept in mind in special circumstances. In general the treatment is surgical, and broadly speaking either the cyst is decompressed by making a permanent opening in its wall (marsupializing the cyst), or the lining is removed in its entirety and the surgical wound primarily repaired.

The aims of the treatment

There are five objectives in the treatment of cysts:

1. To remove the lining, or to enable the patient's body to rearrange the position of the abnormal tissue so that it is eliminated from within the jaw.

2. To do so with the minimum of trauma to the patient, consistent with a successful outcome to the operation.

3. To preserve adjacent important structures such as nerves and healthy teeth.

4. To achieve rapid healing of the operation site.

5. To restore the part to a normal or near normal form and to restore normal function.

Factors to be considered in the choice of operation

The age and physical state of the patient have already been mentioned as factors to be considered. Because most young people are fit and their wounds heal rapidly, and because enlargement of cysts in children is generally rapid, cysts in this age group should receive prompt treatment. Occasionally patients have particular aversions or phobias about certain modes of anaesthesia or treatment. If these cannot be surmounted by explanation, patient management or premedication, a type of treatment other than the ideal may be indicated. Operators vary both in their skill and in their preference for a particular type of operation usually because the chosen technique leads to good results in their hands.

Enucleation of the lining normally removes all the abnormal tissue, and in certain circumstances it may be necessary to provide the pathologist with the entire specimen to facilitate a correct diagnosis. Complete removal of the lining may also be a particularly important feature of the treatment, as in the case of keratocysts.

The surgical accessibility of certain sites is poor, for example the tuberosity region of the maxilla, the lingual aspect of the lower jaw and the ramus of the mandible via the oral cavity. Both the surgical approach and the type of operation may be modified by cysts occurring in these regions.

Where there is a special need to protect or preserve adjacent structures, certain procedures such as the complete enucleation of the lining may be contraindicated, or additional access may be required to ensure that inadvertent damage is avoided.

Enucleation of a cyst and primary closure of the wound leaves a dead space which, as it is in bone, cannot be eliminated by suturing the walls together. Because the clot in the dead space is at risk from infection until it has been replaced by granulation tissue, the larger the bony cavity, the greater the risk. Provided the rules of good flap design and wound closure can be followed, the risk of wound breakdown is small and subsequent clot infection unlikely. Some special methods of managing the dead space are described on p. 39, but for many cases these are unnecessary.

If enucleation and primary closure can be performed, restoration of form and function is not difficult. Where bone loss involves the crest of the ridge, either as a result of the enlargement of the cyst or as a result of the surgery, an unfavourable foundation for a denture may be produced. Consideration can be given under such circumstances to chip bone grafting to improve the denture foundation. Elimination of the cyst and any enclosing bone outside the normal contour of the jaw will both reduce the dead space and restore the facial contour to normal. Restoration of function follows the regeneration of sufficient bone to eliminate the risk of accidental fracture of the jaw and the replacement by prosthetic means of any teeth which have been lost as a result of disease or surgery.

Certain types of cyst require special consideration during treatment.

With a dentigerous cyst under favourable circumstances, it may be possible by marsupializing the cyst and retaining the tooth of origin to allow the latter to erupt into its normal position in the arch. It is reputed that bone does not always regenerate from the margin of a fissural cyst, and for this reason primary closure rather than marsupialization is the preferred treatment. Certainly, it is unwise to open an incisive canal cyst from the palatal aspect and pack it, because this changes the contour of the palate and affects speech. Marsupialization from the labial aspect is unsatisfactory because of poor access when the adjacent teeth are standing, and also because bone regeneration is poor around a cyst of any kind in the front of the maxilla after such treatment. Keratocysts always require special thought and care as to the appropriate treatment, because of their propensity to recur.

Classification of operations for the treatment of benign jaw cysts

While there are only two basic surgical manoeuvres, namely decompression (or marsupialization) and enucleation followed by primary closure of the surgical wound, there are many technical variations. Some of the more important methods are listed below.

Decompression or marsupialization
1. With incomplete removal of the lining
    (a) decompression by opening into the mouth
    (b) decompression by opening into the maxillary sinus or nose
2. With complete removal of the lining
    (a) decompression by opening into the mouth
    (b) decompression by opening into the maxillary sinus or nose

Enucleation with wound closure
1. Without bone grafting
2. With bone grafting
3. Secondary closure after primary decompression

The operative procedure for marsupialization with incomplete removal of the lining

This technique of treating cysts consists of surgically producing a window in the capsular wall to relieve intracystic tension. After this the cystic cavity slowly decreases in size. Ideally the aperture should be as large as possible; if the diameter is small, the aperture may eventually close completely, continuity of the cyst membrane will then be re-established and the cyst will refill and continue to expand.

Marsupialization of cysts of the jaws with retention of part of the lining was advocated by Partsch (1892) and has become known as the Partsch I technique. Although it is a comparatively simple procedure there are certain details of technique which require the operator's attention. Ideally the incision should be placed so that the future edge of the bony opening will be covered by mucosa. It is usual to approach the cyst from the buccal or labial aspect since an alteration to the contour of the palate affects speech; a lingual approach to the mandible is awkward and the resulting opening is restricted in size by the position of the floor of the mouth.

A U-shaped flap is outlined, based on the sulcus. The incision is placed internal to the boundaries of the cyst and just within the anticipated periphery of the bony opening. In some cases a wound designed in this way will be too small to work through, so a larger flap will be raised, but will be trimmed before the cavity is packed and part of it returned to its original site and sutured.

Elevation of the flap is carried out in the subperiosteal plane. This is important in order to conserve the periosteum with its osteogenic potentialities. Furthermore, if the cyst lining has perforated the bone and periosteum is left over the surface it will prove more difficult to separate the lining from the bone edge. To avoid tearing either the flap or any adherent cyst lining, the periosteal elevator must be pressed against the underside of the flap as close as possible to the point of attachment.

Bone removal is normally a straightforward procedure. Where the bone is intact over the cyst, sufficient is removed with a gouge or rosehead bur to permit a pair of rongeur forceps to be employed. Once an opening has been made in the bony wall the lining is separated for some distance from the edge of the opening. Further bone can be removed rapidly with rongeur forceps. The opening in the bone should be made as far as possible in the region normally covered by mucoperiosteum (masticatory mucosa) because the margin will not then contract. Where the teeth have been lost or are due to be extracted, the crest of the ridge must be conserved as a foundation for a denture.

The bone edge is cut back until it lies beneath the border of the surrounding mucoperiosteum, and the cavity should be saucerized as far as this is practical. The adjacent soft tissues can then roll over the rim and come into contact with the cut edge of the lining. The exposed lining should be cut away, flush with the margin of the bony opening. This may be done either with scissors or with a scalpel. If the latter instrument is used the blade is stabbed through the lining, and cutting is done in a direction from within outwards against the bone edge. The detached specimen is sent for section and the cavity gently flushed out.

Any related pulpless teeth either should be extracted or root-filled. If the root filling has not been done prior to the operation, a retrograde root filling should be considered. Any apices of root-filled teeth protrude into the cavity are cut back to just below the inner surface of the lining.

The flap is now turned into the cavity. Suturing of the flap to the cyst lining is not essential provided it can be packed accurately into place. Nor does it matter if the flap overlays the lining, as Wassmund (1935) has shown that epithelium which is covered is rapidly destroyed.

However, if the flap does not adhere rapidly in the right place, an uncomfortable raw area is left to granulate. It is more tidy, therefore, to suture the incised margin of the mucosa to the lining membrane either with 3/0 plain catgut or Dexon. Better haemostasis is also achieved. A round-bodied needle rather than a cutting needle should be used because the cyst membrane is often friable. Care should be taken not to strip the remaining lining from the bony cavity during the suturing process.

The cavity is syringed again with warm sterile saline and lightly packed with 2.5 cm ribbon gauze impregnated with Whitehead's varnish. This pack prevents the contamination of the cavity with food debris and covers any raw wound edges. The composition of Whitehead's varnish is as follows:

    Benzoin 10 g
    Storax 7.5 g
    Balsam of tolu 5 g
    Iodoform 10 g
    Solvent ether to 100 ml

The packing material should first of all be soaked completely in Whitehead's varnish and afterwards surplus fluid is removed by squeezing the roll of gauze in a dry swab. Whitehead's varnish in excess is irritant to the mucosa and therefore the patient's lips should be protected with a wet swab during the process of packing. The insertion of ribbon gauze into the cavity is facilitated by thrusting a straight needle or a silver probe in through to the centre of the roll. An assistant unrolls the ribbon gauze as it is required, while the operator packs it into place with two pairs of non-toothed forceps. The first strip is laid along the floor and the rest inserted systematically in layers running from end to end of the cavity. This arrangement enables the gauze to be withdrawn successfully even if the cavity is undercut. Should there be any raw areas, the single bottom layer rarely sticks tightly, and it can be withdrawn under direct vision after the rest has been removed.

The cut end of the pack is tucked under the rest at one end, and the whole moulded to shape with a damp swab or vaselined gloved finger. In the case of the anaesthetized patient the pack should be firmly sutured to the surrounding tissues to prevent accidental dislodgement with a possible risk of obstruction of the airway during the period of unconsciousness.

The pack is left *in situ* for ten days when it will be found that the line of junction between the lining and the mucosa will have healed (Fig. 6.1). A bung can then be constructed. (Figs. 6.2 and 6.3). The particular indications for a cyst plug are as follows:

1. A bony opening which is small in proportion to the size of the cyst cavity, either for anatomical reasons, or because of the need to avoid damaging adjacent teeth or important structures.

2. An opening where a substantial part of the circumference is com-

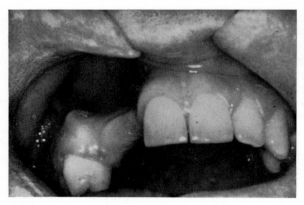

Fig. 6.1 The cavity of a marsupialized cyst in the 432/ area.

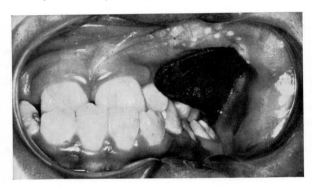

Fig. 6.2 Black gutta-percha bung *in situ* in the patient's mouth. The flange of the plug fits comfortably into the buccal sulcus and the overlying cheek helps to hold the bung in position.

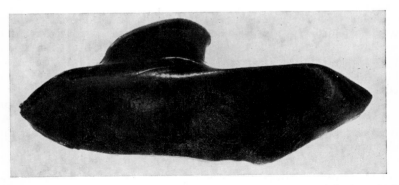

Fig. 6.3 Black gutta-percha bung made to fit the opening into a marsupialized cyst cavity, as used in Fig. 6.2.

posed of sulcus mucosa which is supported on loose connective tissue; i.e., an opening which is *not* surrounded by mucoperiosteum firmly attached to bone. The process of wound contraction can reduce such a defect to a quarter of its size at operation in a period of a few days if the fenestration is not mechanically maintained.

The bung is designed to maintain the patency of the cyst orifice. It should be retentive and should extend into the cavity. However, the projection should never be constructed to reach the full depth of the defect, or it will impede the filling-in process as the cyst cavity decreases in size. Initially it is customary practice to make the plug of a resilient material such as gutta percha to avoid irritation of the healing edges of the wound. Later an acrylic plug can be made, using pink wax moulded directly into the opening both as an impression and as the wax model for the plug. If the patient is wearing a denture, the bung can be attached to an existing plate. In any case the clinician must assure himself that the bung is stable, firmly retained and of a size which is not easily inhaled or swallowed, since it must be worn continuously. The bung must be removed regularly after each meal, the cavity irrigated and the bung replaced. A Higginson's syringe or a glass and rubber socket syringe are suitable for this purpose.

If circumstances do not permit a large portion of the cyst capsule to be removed as, for example, when a full complement of vital teeth is present, then a temporary narrow perforation about 0.5 cm in diameter is made into the cyst cavity. The small size of such an opening makes it easy for scar tissue to occlude the orifice so that further treatment is necessary when the cyst has reduced somewhat in size. The secondary enucleation of such cysts will be dealt with later.

The main advantage of the marsupialization technique is that great surgical skill is not required, and the method is conservative with respect to adjacent important structures. There is virtually no risk of creating an oronasal or oroantral fistula, or of damaging any adjacent major neurovascular bundle. It should be used when there is a risk that enucleation might devitalize many healthy adjacent teeth, the blood supply of which is passing through the cyst capsule. It should also be used when it is hoped that an unerupted tooth involved in a dentigerous cyst will erupt into position. Of course, generally, grossly displaced teeth and teeth in patients over 20 years of age cannot be expected to erupt in this way (Fig. 6.4). There is usually no difficulty with local analgesia since almost all the surgery is confined to the accessible buccal wall of the cyst. Finally, there is little raw tissue exposed at the end of the operation and hence initial healing is rapid and discomfort correspondingly small.

There are three notable disadvantages to the technique. The first is that pathological tissue is left behind. Strictly speaking, it is only when an entire lining can be examined by the pathologist that the surgeon can be certain of the diagnosis and confident that more sinister pathological processes have not been overlooked. In practice, it would seem only

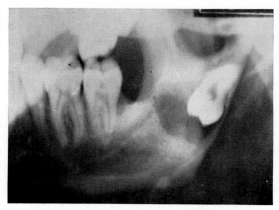

Fig. 6.4 A large dentigerous cyst was marsupialized five years previously. The third molar associated with the cyst was not extracted at the time of operation and is now buried deep in the jaw bone and associated with an area of chronic infection.

remotely possible that a neoplastic change would be so localized that some hint of its presence could not be ascertained on histological examination, provided a respectable biopsy specimen was made available. In any case the cavity is left open and the surface is available for inspection at follow-up visits.

Secondly, if the cavity is large it will take a long time to fill in, and frequently the patient finds this embarrassing. Certainly if rapid progress is not made within the first few months further healing will be very slow indeed (Fig. 6.5). In particular, healing is dilatory in cases of maxillary cysts which have perforated the palatal plate so that the lining is attached

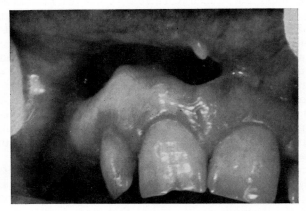

Fig. 6.5 This fissural (globulomaxillary) cyst was marsupialized two years previously but no diminution in size has occurred.

to the palatal mucosa. Indeed they tend to reduce in height but not depth, producing a slit-like cavity which is difficult to clean. (Figs. 6.6 and 6.7).

Thirdly, as indicated above, if only a small opening can be made a cyst plug must be worn.

Operative procedure for marsupialization with complete removal of the lining

The marsupialization of a cyst after complete removal of the lining is similar in most particulars to the previously described operation. When the bony opening has been completed, the entire lining is separated from the cavity and removed. Since the cavity is to be packed, however, the result will not be prejudiced if, as a result of unexpected difficulty in the removal of the lining, some fragments are retained.

As the cavity is to be packed open, any overlapping or excessive tissue is trimmed away from the buccal mucoperiosteal flap with Mayo scissors until the flap sits comfortably in the cavity. It is turned into the cavity to cover part of the bare area of the bone and packed over with 2.5-cm ribbon gauze impregnated with Whitehead's varnish. In a large cavity where it might be feared that the pack will stick to the walls, a layer of Surgicel or tulle gras can be applied before the ribbon gauze pack.

The cavity is repacked with ribbon gauze at ten days postoperatively, and a bung fitted where necessary at the end of three weeks when the cavity will be granulating.

Whilst the method is still a simple one, a little more expertise is required than when the deep part of the lining is left. One advantage of the technique is that pathological tissue is not left behind. Another is that reputedly the cavity becomes smaller more rapidly when it fills with granulation tissue from all aspects and the period before complete epithelialization is delayed. Whether this proposition is correct is difficult to substantiate, due to the varying speed with which cysts fill in after marsupialization with retention of part of the lining.

Beyond these two advantages, the technique has most of the disadvantages of both marsupialization with retention of part of the lining and enucleation with primary closure and, moreover, without the benefit of rapid restoration of the normal anatomy of the ridge, which is a feature of primary closure of the wound.

One major difficulty which can follow enucleation and packing of a cyst in the maxilla is a tear in the nasal or antral mucosa, which may result from difficulty in separating the cyst lining from these structures. Such tears are difficult to repair. The mucosa needs mobilization sufficient to permit everting horizontal mattress sutures to be inserted. Holes also should be drilled from the bony cavity through to the palatal aspect and a buccal flap of adequate length mobilized, advanced and sutured through these holes to cover the repair. The pack will hold the flap down on to the underlying tissues. Wassmund (1935) advocates that in such

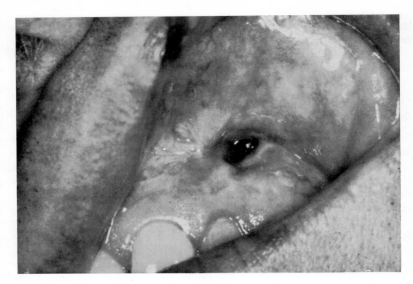

Fig. 6.6

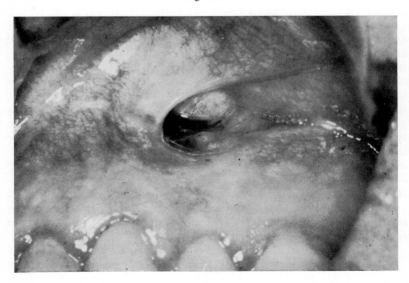

Fig. 6.7

Figs. 6.6 and 6.7 These two large cysts were marsupialized and in neither case, despite prolonged observation, has the cyst cavity been obliterated entirely. This is often the end result of marsupialization except in the young patient, and in the examples illustrated it is unlikely that further natural contraction of the defects will occur.

cases the lining should be left over the mucosa of the respiratory passage and reinforced with a buccal flap as described. The covered epithelium is soon destroyed and causes no problems.

Decompression by opening into the maxillary sinus or nose

The many technical variations of this method which were developed from the latter part of the last century onwards have been reviewed by Seward and Seward (1969). Briefly, the operation is valuable for very large cysts of the maxilla which entirely occupy a maxillary sinus, and perhaps also one or both inferior meati of the nose.

A satisfactory operative technique is as follows. An incision is made around the necks of the teeth or along the crest of the ridge from the tuberosity round to the lateral incisor region on the other side and then up into the buccal sulcus. Where the anterior teeth are to be retained the incision can be taken up into the sulcus just distal to the canine and then forward through the vestibular mucosa (Wassmund 1935).

The palatal flap is raised because where a cortical perforation exists, it is easier to elevate the mucoperiosteum from the cyst lining than to dissect the latter from the periosteum through the buccal wound. Care should be taken not to damage the palatine vessels or this will affect healing. Elevation of the buccal flap begins over sound bone to achieve the correct subperiosteal plane of dissection.

Commonly, an opening of sufficient size already exists in the bone on the lateral aspect of the maxilla, and before enucleation of the lining is started the whole periphery of such a perforation should be uncovered. Any surgical removal of bone found necessary should be performed with caution so as not to weaken the attachment of the alveolar process, and it may be prudent to extract first those teeth which must be lost. Any teeth the apices of which are denuded of bone by the cyst must be either root filled or extracted.

Extractions some time prior to the main operation are best avoided, because perforation of the cyst followed by decompression and subacute infection follows. Similarly, extractions in the early postoperative period lead to oroantral fistulae.

The whole cyst lining is removed, so that later the cavity walls will be covered by a normal ciliated and mucus-secreting epithelium regenerating from the respiratory mucosa. Care is taken to dissect the lining out in one piece to ensure complete removal.

The partition between the cyst cavity and the deformed maxillary sinus is breached towards the zygomatic extension to avoid the risk of damage to the infraorbital nerve or the floor of the orbit. The whole partition should be removed by inserting a periosteal elevator or finger into the sinus cavity and levering gently downwards. If the antral mucosa can be retained as a flap it can be packed against the bony wall of the cyst partially to cover it. Once blood clot has filled the lining to the bone the pack is removed and the incision is closed.

A small, temporary intranasal antrostomy is fashioned and the new combined cyst-sinus cavity drained with a 0.75 cm diameter sterile polythene tube. A pair of angled nasal forceps are introduced through the nostril and through the antrostomy. The pointed end of the drain is grasped with the forceps inside the cavity and drawn outwards through the nose. The nasal end is cut off short and sewn securely to the ala of the nose. The drain is necessary to prevent a haematoma developing postoperatively and creating tension at the suture line.

The buccal periosteum is divided in the usual way above the level of the sulcus and the flap advanced to cover any sockets. The wound is closed carefully and without tension.

The advantages of the technique are mainly those associated with primary closure of the oral wound: namely, that there is no large cavity leading off from the mouth of which the patient is aware and which has to be kept free of food debris. Restoration of the normal anatomy of the maxillary sinus and nose is more rapid than after simple enucleation and closure. However, should there be any wound breakdown, an oroantral fistula will be created. In most cases, the risk of wound breakdown is less than after enucleation and primary closure, since the cavity is drained and tension on the suture line is less likely in the event of postoperative oozing.

Operative procedure for enucleation of a cyst and primary wound closure (Figs. 6.8–6.18)

This surgical procedure leaves the surgical opening into the cyst cavity covered by a mucoperiosteal flap and the space filled with blood clot which eventually organizes to form normal bone. The method is often called the Partsch II technique (Partsch 1910). Undoubtedly this is the most satisfactory method of treatment of a cyst, for the patient is spared the inconvenience of a large cavity in the mouth which requires frequent irrigation with a syringe over a long period. As soon as the incision heals the patient is no longer troubled, and from the surgeon's point of view the method avoids tedious postoperative measures, such as packing and irrigation of the wound and the fitting of a cyst plug. Following primary closure it is impossible to observe the healing of the cyst by direct vision and, therefore, it is necessary to have follow-up radiographs of the area at regular intervals to observe the progress of bone regeneration and eventual obliteration of the defect by normal bone.

There are three circumstances in which this method of treatment may be contraindicated. These are:

1. A large cyst in the mandible for which the necessary surgical access would so weaken the jaw that a fracture might result. In this type of case it is advisable at first to marsupialize through a limited opening and, when sufficient bone has reformed, secondary enucleation of the tissue lining the cavity is carried out followed by primary closure to hasten healing.

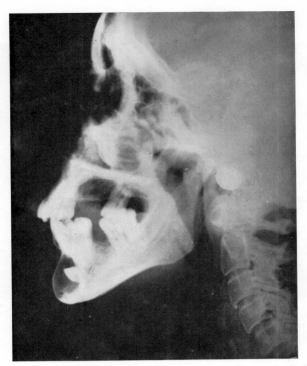

Fig. 6.8 True lateral radiograph showing a dentigerous cyst in the lower incisor region.

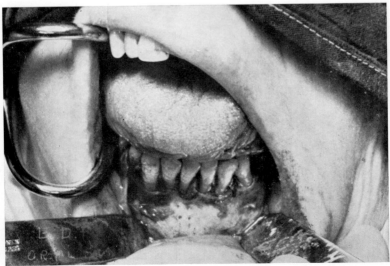

Fig. 6.9 The surgical exposure for the enucleation of the cyst shown in Fig. 6.8 was made by taking the incision around the necks of the standing teeth. The cyst sac is covered with a layer of bone.

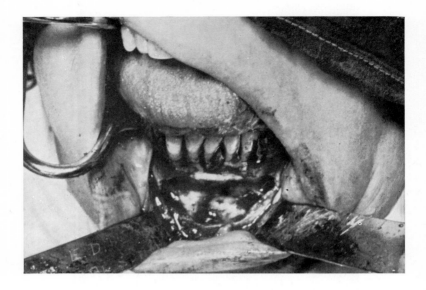

Fig. 6.10 The overlying cortical plate shown in Fig. 6.9 has been removed to expose the cyst margins.

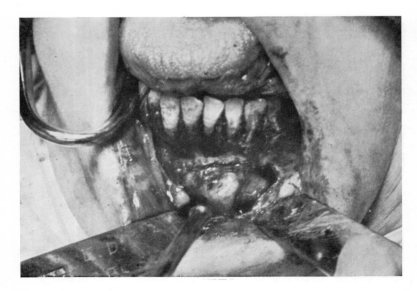

Fig. 6.11 The cyst capsule shown in Fig. 6.10 has been detached from the enclosing bone, and the canine tooth still adherent to cyst tissue has been elevated from its socket.

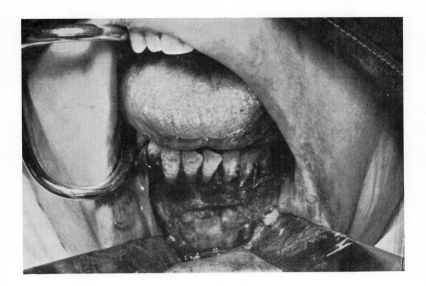

Fig. 6.12 The cyst and its attached canine tooth as shown in Fig. 6.11 have been removed revealing the bony defect.

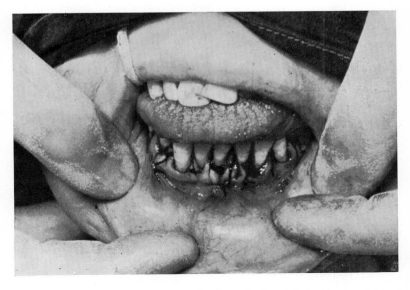

Fig. 6.13 Primary closure of the cyst cavity shown in Fig. 6.12 by interrupted sutures passing from the lingual to the buccal side through the interdental spaces.

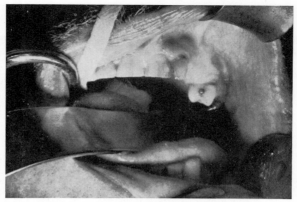

Fig. 6.14 Preoperative view of a residual periodontal cyst in the /34 area.

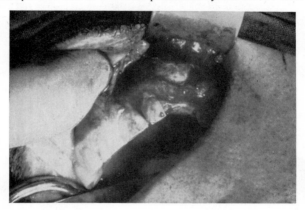

Fig. 6.15 Surgical exposure for the removal of the cyst shown in Fig. 6.14. The overlying soft tissues have been separated from the cyst capsule and retracted.

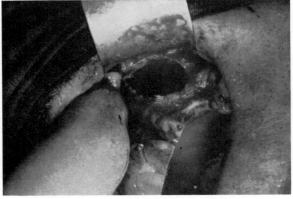

Fig. 6.16 The cyst shown in Fig. 6.15 has now been dissected out, leaving an empty bony cavity.

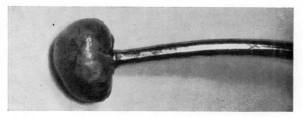

Fig. 6.17 The intact cyst specimen which was taken from the bony space shown in Fig. 6.16 is held by the sucker nozzle.

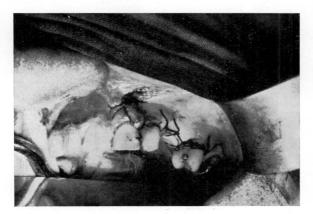

Fig. 6.18 Primary closure of the residual cavity shown in Fig. 6.17.

In practice surprisingly large cysts can be enucleated safely by the experienced operator. However, if wound breakdown supervenes with infection and sequestration of part of the bony wall, a pathological fracture can result. Prompt drainage of the cavity should be carried out if infection does supervene. Fracture may well occur postoperatively as a result of injudicious action on the part of the patient, and a radiograph early in the postoperative period is a necessary safeguard to prevent the patient attributing the injury to the operator.

Where there is a preoperative crack or an overt fracture, gentle marsupialization with the insertion of a pack may immobilize the fracture better than transosseous wires inserted into thin bone. Mandibular-maxillary fixation is of course required. Whenever there is a danger of fracture through a cyst cavity the preoperative construction of suitable splints is a sensible precaution. Indeed, when operating on a large mandibular cyst where there is a possible risk of fracture occurring, it may be prudent to splint the jaws preoperatively as a precautionary measure until some bone regeneration has taken place (Figs. 6.19 and 6.20). The

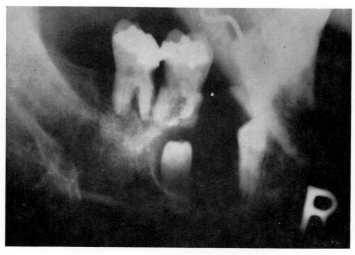

Fig. 6.19 Dentigerous cyst containing 54/ in relation to lower border of mandible.

possibility should be explained to the patient, but with a reassurance that all proper care will be taken.

2. A cyst which involves the apices of one or more healthy teeth in such a way that the blood supply to the pulp passes through the capsule of the lining. Stripping out the cyst sac will result in necrosis of the pulps of the teeth concerned. If it is desired to conserve the pulps of such teeth and avoid extraction or root canal therapy, the cyst should be treated by marsupialization.

3. A dentigerous cyst in a young person which is preventing the tooth concerned and perhaps others from erupting. Marsupialization is usually followed by satisfactory eruption of the involved teeth, although orthodontic treatment may be needed subsequently to ensure that they achieve their normal position in the arch (Fig. 6.21).

Before operating upon a cyst involving the roots of teeth, it is important to decide provisionally which teeth are to be conserved, and which are useless and should be extracted. It is also prudent to consider if the lining will be in any way difficult to enucleate. The lining can be expected to be adherent if:

(a) The cyst has already been decompressed by the extraction of a tooth, the development of a sinus or the need for a drainage incision in its wall. In these circumstances bone will be growing in towards the fibrous capsule.

(b) The cyst has eroded the cortex and the lining is in contact with the periosteum, particularly the thin mucoperiosteum of the maxillary sinus or nose.

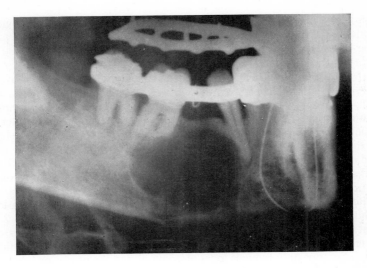

Fig. 6.20 Cyst shown in Fig. 6.19 enucleated and 54/ removed without causing a mandibular fracture. The mandible has been immobilized as a precautionary measure.

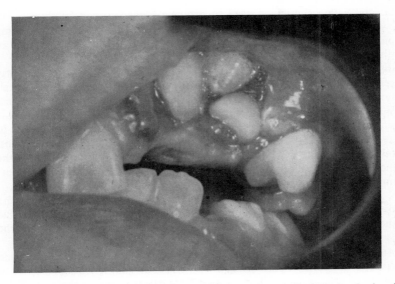

Fig. 6.21 A dentigerous cyst containing three teeth was marsupialized. The involved teeth are now erupting, but orthodontic treatment will be necessary in the future.

C

(c) The lining is attached to the periodontal membrane of adjacent teeth.

The lining may also be friable:

(a) If the cyst has been grossly infected.

(b) If the lining is very thin, as, for example, in the case of keratocyst.

A preoperative decision on these matters and hence the type of operation is proper, because the flap design for enucleation and primary closure is different from that used for marsupialization. The incision should be of adequate length to give good surgical exposure and designed so that the edge of the flap will rest on a good, sound, bony margin at the end of the operation. Mucoperiosteal flaps cannot be closed in layers, and if the incision crosses the cystic cavity, postoperative breakdown of the suture line is almost inevitable.

Before marking the incision the area should be infiltrated with a local analgesic solution containing a vasoconstrictor such as lignocaine 2 per cent with 1:80 000 adrenaline, or prilocaine (Citanest) in a 3 per cent concentration which contains felypressin 0.03 i.u/ml. This preliminary procedure not only reduces local bleeding during the operation, but if the local anaesthetic fluid has insinuated itself between the cyst lining and the overlying soft tissues, the tissue planes can be identified easily and the cyst exposed without the risk of an inadvertent perforation. If a general anaesthetic is being administered, a solution of adrenaline 1:200 000 in normal saline should be used to produce local vasoconstriction.

The incision is made well wide of the anticipated surgical bony opening and carried down on to bone so that the correct subperiosteal plane of dissection is established. If the patient is edentulous the incision is directed along the crest of the ridge (Figs. 6.22–6.25), but if teeth are present the incision line is taken around the necks of adjoining teeth buccally, lingually or palatally, depending upon the position of the cyst. Whenever possible a buccal approach is preferable because of the superior visibility and access. It is important while raising the flap to avoid unnecessary damage to it and, in particular, to its margins, otherwise healing will be impaired. The tissues on the opposite side of the incision are also raised 3 to 4 mm so as to provide a cuff for easy suturing.

After the mucoperiosteal flap has been raised, it will depend upon the size of the cyst whether a hard bony prominence, a thin, compressible shell of expanded bone, or a fluctuant swelling due to destruction of the overlying cortex is found at the site of the lesion.

If the bone covering the cyst is intact, a window should be made through the cortical plate using a bur, chisel or gouge, taking care not to puncture or tear the wall of the cyst. It is easier to define the margins of the cyst if the membrane is not ruptured, and enucleation is simplified because the lining strips easily from the bony cavity as the fluid content of the sac is compressed. The opening can then be enlarged with a pair of Jansen–Middleton bone nibblers until it is sufficiently large that separa-

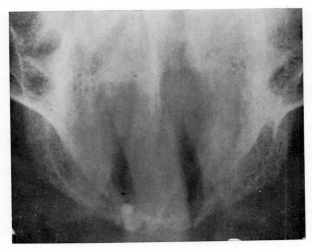

Fig. 6.22 An occlusal radiograph showing a moderate-sized maxillary cyst.

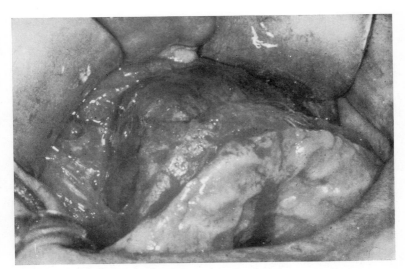

Fig. 6.23 The cyst illustrated in Fig. 6.22 has been enucleated.

tion and removal of the lining will not be too difficult. It is helpful to separate the lining progressively from the margin of the bony opening before using the bone nibblers as this avoids tears in the wall of the sac. It also makes it easier to judge the position of the cavity and to avoid damage to important neighbouring structures.

If a thin layer of fragmented bone is present on reflecting the flap, the

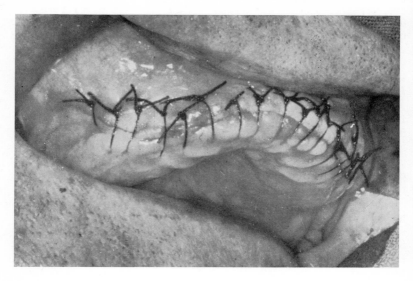

Fig. 6.24 The suture line following primary closure of the cyst cavity seen in Fig. 6.23.

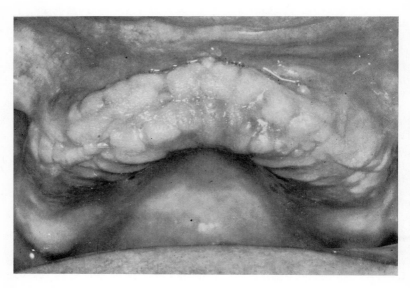

Fig. 6.25 The sutures shown in Fig. 6.24 were removed on the tenth postoperative day.

numerous small pieces should be peeled off the underlying cyst membrane with a pair of Fickling's forceps. The edges of the exposed bony cavity should then be trimmed back with bone nibblers. When part of the lining of the cyst is visible after elevation of the flap, the lining is separated from the bone edge and the opening enlarged with Jansen–Middleton forceps as before.

The attached lining is gently eased away from the bony cavity with a Howarth's periosteal elevator, the broad curved end of which is pressed firmly against the surface of the bone. Depending on the size and position of the cyst, Howarth's periosteal elevator, curved Warwick James root elevators, a large binangled spoon excavator or a Mitchell's trimmer are other instruments which are useful for separating the lining. In all cases the edge of the instrument is applied to the bone so that the concave surface of the blade faces the lining. Often, it is best to begin the dissection from before back or from a point nearest the crest of the ridge. Great care should be taken not to rupture the lining of the cyst as the instrument is advanced, and this can be avoided by ensuring that the plane of separation is correct. Often the entire cyst sac can be removed cleanly from its bony cavity without bursting it, but, even if the cyst is punctured, careful manipulation should succeed in freeing the lining from its attachment and ensure a complete removal. A thick cyst lining is obviously easier to enucleate than a thin-walled sac such as that of the keratocyst type. If the undersurface of the cyst lining is in close relationship to the inferior dental neurovascular bundle or has displaced that structure, meticulous dissection is essential to release the cyst from its attachments while avoiding damage to the nerve and vessels. In general it is safer to separate the lining by working along the length of the nerve, rather than by approaching it from the side. Caution is also necessary when cyst tissue is in contact with the lining of the nose or the maxillary sinus. The lining usually adheres firmly to the mucoperiosteum of the nose and maxillary sinuses, and if possible it should be retracted so that a dissecting pressure may be applied accurately to the lining at its point of separation from respiratory mucoperiosteum. If this is not done either the cyst lining or the mucoperiosteum will be torn. In the latter case a nasal or antral perforation may be produced.

Aspiration of the cyst contents so that the sac collapses may aid visualization of an adherent area. Sometimes dissection is aided by first retracting the cyst lining with the Howarth's periosteal elevator and then using a blunt sucker nozzle gently to separate the cyst from its soft tissue covering and bony bed.

Another manoeuvre is to push a gauze swab held in a pair of non-toothed forceps gradually into the interval between the lining and the wall of the cavity in its deepest part. If at any stage difficulty is experienced the operator should direct his efforts elsewhere, so mobilizing the tissues to the maximum before the more difficult part is tackled.

When the cyst lining has been removed the bony cavity should be irrigated and then thoroughly inspected after drying its surface with a swab. If the dissection has been successful there should not be any residual cyst remnants, but if pieces of pathological tissue remain they should be removed with mosquito artery forceps. Under no circumstances, however, should the cyst lining be grasped initially with a pair of artery forceps and pulled out. Forcible traction may result in injury to adjacent structures (such as the neurovascular bundle) and the tearing of the cyst lining so that enucleation is more difficult and the specimen less suitable for microscopic examination.

If the neurovascular bundle is exposed it should be examined to confirm that it has not been severed or traumatized. When either nasal mucosa or antral lining is visible after removal of cyst tissue, the mucous membrane should be inspected to ascertain that it has remained imperforate. Any openings into the nose or maxillary sinus should be repaired carefully with everting horizontal mattress sutures. If an effective repair is possible, primary closure of the oral wound can still be carried out.

The cavity should be inspected also to ensure that the apices of all related teeth are covered with bone and that the blood supply of their pulps is intact. Any teeth with apices denuded of bone should be either root-filled or extracted.

The cyst cavity should now be packed with a dry swab until bleeding is arrested. The main cause of breakdown of the suture line following primary closure is the development of tension as a result of haematoma formation outside the bony cavity. This is caused by a brisk delayed haemorrhage into the bony defect after the initial control of bleeding at the end of operation. Once the flap is raised from the broad surface of bone surrounding the bony opening into the cyst cavity the effect of a valve-like closure is lost. A tenuous union of wound edge to wound edge only can develop during the early stages of healing and this is insufficient to resist the tensions which develop as a result of facial movements. It has been found that if bleeding is stopped by pressure with a dry gauze swab before suturing the reflected flap back into its correct position, sufficient blood will subsequently seep into the operative area to fill the cavity. This practice ensures the retention of an amount of blood clot consistent with satisfactory organization, and is compatible with new bone formation later.

In mandibular cysts the amount of dead space and the tendency to liquefaction and breakdown of the blood clot with failure of organization can be minimized by trimming the bone margins of the defect until it is saucerized. In addition to eliminating part of the dead space, this measure allows the buccal tissues to collapse into the dead space. The judicious application of a pressure pack can help this process. In the upper jaw it is not advisable to attempt this manoeuvre for it could cause deformity of either the denture-bearing ridge or the facial contour. Experience has shown that it is possible to carry out successful primary closure of the largest cyst provided that excessive bleeding is prevented. The introduction of drains to relieve tension is not necessary.

In order to obliterate the cavity following enucleation various filling materials have been suggested for packing into the defect prior to closure of the wound. Mostly these are forms of haemostatic resorbable sponge, some of which may be soaked in a solution containing an antibiotic, in the hope that they will form a scaffolding into which granulation tissue can migrate should the clot liquefy before this can happen. There is no evidence that such a scaffold is necessary or better than normal clot, and the probable benefit comes from the haemostatic properties of these materials so that the clot is confined to the bony cavity and tension on the flaps is reduced. On the other hand, if wound breakdown does occur, an unresorbed and infected foreign body has to be removed instead of an infected clot which could be syringed out. Autografts of cancellous bone are more effective, but it is questionable whether these are justifiable.

The empty cyst cavity should be gently irrigated with warm normal saline and the flap sutured back into position using interrupted silk sutures. The sutures should remain in situ for ten days, and the patient should be given prophylactic antibiotic therapy for a four-day period postoperatively.

It is feasible to remove infected cysts in this manner and to carry out primary closure, provided that the infection is clinically quiescent and there has not been a recent acute exacerbation. The infection exists primarily within the cyst lining, and after the sac has been removed the cavity should be copiously irrigated with warm saline to remove any contamination from spilt cyst contents. The incision is closed in the usual manner and the use of a prophylactic antibiotic prevents breakdown of the blood clot due to secondary infection.

Should the wound edges of a large cyst separate postoperatively no great harm is done, for by this time part of the enclosed clot is usually organized. The remaining space is irrigated to remove any unorganized elements of clot and loosely packed with 2.5-cm ribbon gauze which has been soaked in Whitehead's varnish. The pack is left in situ for ten days to allow the residual cavity to granulate, after which it will heal rapidly in the manner of a cyst formally treated by enucleation and packing.

Enucleation of a cyst from the palatal aspect

Occasionally a cyst enlarges entirely towards the palatal aspect and an approach from this direction is indicated. As such a cyst increases in size, it displaces the roots of the adjacent vital teeth in a buccal direction and their neurovascular bundles lie in the buccal bone. Under these circumstances a surgical approach from the buccal aspect not only provides poor access, but may damage the blood supply to the pulps of the adjacent teeth.

Access to the apices of anterior teeth in order to place a retrograde root filling is poor, so any pulpless tooth must be root-filled prior to the operation. Unless it is proposed to raise a buccal flap as well as a palatal one, a palatal approach is inappropriate where teeth are to be extracted as the palatal mucosa cannot be advanced to cover the socket.

A palatal flap is raised and the opening in the bone suitably enlarged. The lining is enucleated and any local expansions of bone which have altered the normal bony contour are nibbled away. Naturally, any bone excision must not approach too close to the necks of the teeth or no adequate shelf of bone will remain on which the flap can rest. After haemostasis has been assured the flap is sutured back into place by the usual method of interdental suturing. A previously prepared acrylic palatal plate which is retained by cribs on suitable posterior teeth is lined in the region of the original swelling with soft, black gutta percha so as to correct the contour of the fitting surface to that of a normal palate. The plate is seated in position and will prevent distention of the palatal flap by a haematoma.

The plate should be removed and cleaned after meals and then replaced from the second postoperative day onwards. At 14 days postoperatively the sutures are removed and the plate discarded. By this technique a direct approach can be made to the cyst, and by the time primary wound healing has occurred, palatal contour has been restored to normality.

Enucleation and primary closure with bone grafting

It is known that grafting with cancellous bone can be successfully performed through oral wounds. It is obvious, therefore, that chip grafting of cyst cavities should have been tried. However, it has been adequately shown by Killey *et al.* (1966, 1970) and Kramer *et al.* (1968 a, b, c) that anorganic bone and similar processed and stored heterogenous bone does not act as a graft, and indeed seems to impede natural bone regeneration although it may perform a function in preserving space.

The use of homologous bone implies the existence of a bone bank to which the operator has access. Sterile healthy bone removed at operation, for example lengths of rib, or suitable cadaver bone, is freeze dried and stored until required. If the operator does not have access to a bone bank, autogenous bone must be used which adds to the extent of the operation. However, cancellous bone together with bone marrow, which also has osteogenic properties (Boyne 1970) can be obtained readily through quite small wounds over the crest of the ilium. Although in recent years the importance of the marrow component of these grafts has been explained, there would seem to be little difference between the grafts and the cancellous chips used by Mowlem (1944) Scott *et al.* (1949) and Flint (1964). Where grafting is indicated, autogenous bone gives the best results if a second wound is not a major consideration.

Advantages

The obvious advantage is maintenance of bone contour, particularly where the cyst involves a future denture-bearing area. There will also be a more rapid increase in strength of the bone as the graft consolidates and this may be of particular importance in the case of large cysts involving the mandible. In the case of large cysts, with the exception of keratocysts, the follow-up period will also be shorter because the bone cavity will be more rapidly obliterated.

The most obvious disadvantage is the added difficulties which result from the presence of infected bone fragments where wound breakdown occurs. The risk of failure is, in fact, greater than where grafts are placed after resection of a segment of mandible, because of the greater difficulty in effecting a watertight wound closure. Considerable surgical skill is therefore required. What is more, large cysts are not infrequently chronically infected and copious wound irrigation is necessary after removal of the lining. Careful surgical judgement is essential to appraise the importance of such wound contamination. Clearly where grafting is contemplated there is much to be said in favour of homologous bone grafts.

It is in the maxilla, probably, that the question of an impaired denture foundation is most likely to arise. Whether the grafting of a large cyst involving the antrum would be likely to delay remodelling of the antral cavity seems not to be known.

Against the indications for the operation is the speed with which bone can regenerate after more simple procedures, although of course such regeneration will not add to the external contour of the jaw.

Secondary enucleation and wound closure

The indications for secondary enucleation and wound closure have been mentioned previously. Once sufficient bone has been deposited to cover and protect the particular structures at risk the lining may be enucleated and flaps raised to close over the defect.

Once a cyst has been decompressed for some time the lining will be thickened and made stiff by an increased layer of fibrous tissue. The boundary between capsule and bony cavity will become irregular with spicules of bone penetrating into the capsule. Thus enucleation may be far from easy. Once the cavity has been opened to the mouth, and particularly if the opening is limited in extent, infected debris will tend to accumulate in it. Removal of the lining will of course remove the epithelium and its surface contamination.

It is next necessary to prepare a flap to cover the defect. This is usually best done by lateral displacement of the mucoperiosteum from one side of the opening, rather than by an attempt to advance sulcus and cheek mucosa. It is important that the flap should be wide enough to extend generously beyond the bony opening and that its margin should rest without tension against the opposing wound edge.

Follow-up

All cyst patients should be followed up postoperatively. Both clinical inspection of the site of surgery and radiographs of the affected bone are needed at regular intervals. Once soft tissue healing is complete after a primary closure of the wound, the radiographic examination assumes greater importance than if the cyst has been marsupialized. Follow-up should continue until the anatomy of the part has returned as closely as possible to its preoperative state. Visits at 1, 3, 6, 12 and 24 months after primary wound healing is complete is a reasonable schedule after the treatment of a sizeable cyst.

Any teeth adjacent to the surgical field should be tested for pulp sensation as soon as the sutures have been removed. Those which do not respond should be re-tested and observed closely. When it is thought that this sign indicates pulpal necrosis, appropriate treatment should be initiated.

Where there has been a change in conductivity of a major nerve adjacent to the cyst, this should be monitored until recovery is noted, or until a stage is reached where further improvement seems unlikely.

The mechanical aspects of cyst treatment in relationship to recurrence

From the viewpoint of the operating surgeon, the feature that distinguishes a benign lesion from one which is locally infiltrative is the fact that its periphery can be distinguished with certainty at operation, and, therefore, that it can be separated with confidence from the surrounding normal tissue. Even if the lesion is classified as benign by other criteria, if the periphery is not readily recognized at operation then part of the lesion may be left behind and a recurrence is certain.

Some neoplasms infiltrate the adjacent normal tissues and hence do not possess a periphery that can be clearly distinguished by observation at operation. A margin of apparently normal tissue must be removed around all aspects of the mass if complete excision is to be ensured. The size of this margin is arbitrary, but a knowledge of the behaviour of similar neoplasms in others and the effect of the neoplasm in the particular patient is judged by what is seen in the biopsy, and may guide the operator. When the type of tissue at the periphery of the tumour varies, the degree to which the neoplasm is capable of infiltrating them may be known and a different thickness of tissue may be removed over different aspects of the lesion. In general, a generous margin will ensure complete removal, but will do more damage to the patient. A further judgement balancing these two aspects is necessary. Ameloblastomas are examples of cystic lesions of the jaws which behave in this way.

In some cases it is known that cells shed from the surface of a neoplasm are capable of surviving as local grafts; this is 'seeding' of the neoplasm. Where this is a possibility, surgery must be conducted in such a way that the surgeon does not cut into any part of the neoplasm.

Furthermore, where a surface is exposed by ulceration or by biopsy, every care must be taken to prevent the transfer of cells from that surface into the tissues. There is substantial evidence that ameloblastomas can 'seed' in this fashion and some suggestion that keratocysts may, on occasion, behave in a similar manner.

Certain conditions are multicentric in origin. This term implies that several similar lesions arise simultaneously or at different times in a particular region, and each is thought to have originated independently of the other. A single predisposing factor links the lesions and accounts for their occurrence in this way. Keratocysts are sometimes multicentric, particularly in cases of the multiple cyst—basal cell naevus syndrome. Some recurrences of keratocysts are explained on the grounds of their multicentric origin. Where the susceptible tissue can be removed with ease at the time when the first lesion is removed, the subsequent development of new lesions may be avoided. An example of the use of this manoeuvre is the performance of a lip shave for a 'lip at risk' at the same time that a wedge resection of a carcinoma is performed.

Malignant lesions which not only infiltrate into adjacent tissue but also metastasize present yet more problems for the surgeon who would seek to treat them by excision. The latter are outside the terms of reference of this book.

For surgery to be successful, careful thought must be given to the behaviour of the particular cyst under consideration. This is the biological aspect of the problem. Next, it must be decided what operative procedures are necessary to remove the cyst and to ensure against recurrence. These are the anatomical and technical aspects of the problem. Then, the outcome if no treatment were undertaken together with the degree of morbidity which might result from the proposed surgery must be considered – this is the moral side of the problem. These topics are considered further, where appropriate, when the different types of cyst are considered and particularly when keratocysts are discussed (p. 62).

REFERENCES

Boyne, P. J. (1956) *J. Oral Surg.*, **15**, 236.
Boyne, P. J. (1970) *Clin. Orthop.*, **73**, 199.
Flint, M. (1964) *Brit J. plast. Surg.*, **17**, 184.
Killey, H. C., Kramer, I. R. H. & Wright, H. C. (1966) *Archs. oral Biol*, **11**, 1117.
Killey, H. C., Kramer, I. R. H. & Wright, H. C. (1970) *Archs. oral Biol.*, **15**, 33.
Kramer, I. R. H., Killey, H. C. & Wright, H. C. (1968a) *Aus. dent. J.*, **13**, 17.
Kramer, I. R. H., Killey, H. C. & Wright, H. C. (1968b) *Archs. oral Biol.* **13**, 1095.
Kramer, I. R. H., Killey, H. C. & Wright, H. C. (1968c), *Archs. oral Biol.*, **13**, 1263
Mowlem, R. (1944) *Lancet*, **2**, 746.
Partsch, C., (1892) *Deutsche Mschr. Zahnheilkunde.*, **7**, 19.
Partsch, C., (1910) *Deutsche Mschr. Zahnheilkunde*, **28**, 252.
Scott, W., Peterson, R. C. and Grant, S. (1949) *J. Bone Jt. Surg.*, **31A**, 860.
Seward, M. H. and Seward, G. R. (1969) *Brit. J. oral Surg.*, **6**, 149.
Wassmund, M. (1935) *Lehrbuch der praktischen Chirurgie des Mundes und der Kiefer*, Bard 1. Leipzig: Meusser.

7. Odontogenic Keratocysts

At one time, both dentigerous cysts and primordial cysts were classified as follicular cysts, the latter being referred to as simple follicular cysts. In 1945, Robinson published a classification which gained wide acceptance, so popularizing the term 'primordial cyst'. At the same time the concept was spread that such cysts resulted from degeneration of the stellate reticulum of a tooth germ; that is, cystic degeneration at a stage before the dental hard tissues are deposited. According to Harris (1974), this idea has its roots in a monograph by Magitot (1872). The latter stated that certain follicular cysts develop prior to the formation of any dental hard tissues, but after the enamel organ has been formed. Magitot distinguished between 'neogenic' or periosteal dental cysts and follicular cysts. The latter he classified according to the stage of development at which the tooth germ was disturbed.

Seward (1963) redefined primordial cysts as cysts arising from odontogenic epithelial cells which had not taken a direct part in the development of a tooth and, therefore, did not bear a close physical relationship to a tooth. Kramer (1974) also took the view that primordial cysts can develop from various parts of the odontogenic epithelium, and pointed out the difficulties which stem from relating their origin to an enamel organ — the need, firstly, to postulate that cysts which arise in an area with no missing teeth develop from supernumerary tooth germs, and secondly, to recognize that they are uncommon in regions where supernumerary teeth are frequently found. Toller (1967) took the view that the tooth primordium is the dental lamina and that primordial cysts are derived from undifferentiated dental lamina.

More recently a fundamental division of odontogenic cysts has emerged, separating them into those arising from the cell rests of Malassez from the reduced enamel epithelium, and those from the cell rests of the dental lamina (Main, 1970a, Harris 1974). Those arising from the dental lamina are thought, in the main, to have the keratocyst type of lining; they include the primordial cyst.

The term keratocyst was introduced by Philipsen in 1956 and is based upon the histological appearance of the lining. Shear (1960) sets out the histological criteria as follows:

1. A regular, thin lining of stratified squamous epithelium, with no rete pegs.

2. The presence of a keratinized or parakeratinized layer on the surface of the epithelium. Keratin is frequently present within the cyst cavity.

3. A relative absence of inflammatory cell infiltration.

4. The presence of columnar basal cells with either pyknotic or vesicular nuclei.

'Keratocyst', therefore, is a term used by the histopathologist. As has been mentioned in the chapter on dentigerous cysts (Chapter 8), extrafollicular dentigerous cysts also have the keratocyst lining. Extrafollicular dentigerous cysts resemble primary dentigerous cysts both in their clinical and radiographical features. It is at operation that the difference may be appreciated for the first time, and only if the relationship of the tooth crown to the cyst cavity is examined. In some cases the keratinized surface of the lining gives it a shimmering, fish-scale appearance and the contents may be creamy white, as is usual in the case of keratocysts. Thus 'primordial cyst' and 'extrafollicular dentigerous cyst' are clinical terms describing the clinical, radiographic and operative findings. Keratocyst is a histopathological term based upon the type of lining which is common to both.

Extrafollicular dentigerous cysts almost certainly arise from the epithelial glands of Serres, i.e. the remnants of the dental lamina close above the tooth follicle, so that the contention that keratocysts are cysts arising from the dental lamina is not challenged. Most dentigerous cysts seen in the multiple cyst syndrome are of the extrafollicular type.

Main (1970b) introduced another terminology for these cysts. He subdivided primordial cysts into the classical 'replacement' variety, where the cyst develops at the site of a tooth missing from the permanent series, the 'envelopmental' type which encloses an entire tooth and which presumably is similar to the extrafollicular dentigerous cyst, the 'extraneous' type which arises remote from any teeth and the 'collateral' type which arises in the healthy periodontal membrane of a vital tooth. The latter type is considered in Chapter 8 as the developmental periodontal cyst.

Primordial cysts may be unilocular or multilocular, whereas extrafollicular dentigerous cysts are usually radiographically unilocular. Indeed, the latter may be unilocular even when the cyst impedes the eruption of two adjacent molars which may be seen with crown facing crown within the one bony cavity. Mostly keratocysts have a thin lining, but on occasions the lining is very thick and lined by an epithelium with a thick layer of orthokeratinized cells on its surface. Daughter cysts lined by a similar epithelium may be found in the capsule of such a cyst, some of which are small and fail to indent the wall of the containing bony cavity. Once a keratocyst has been infected many of its characteristics, including the thinness of the lining, tend to be lost.

Bernier (1955) contended that primordial cysts were rare, for he found only three cases in a series of 400 cysts of all types in the files of the Armed Forces Institute of Pathology. Support for that view comes from Shafer *et al.* (1963), who stated that these lesions constitute the least common variety of odontogenic cyst, but Shear (1960) after studying 22 cases of primordial cyst considered that they probably form about 10 per cent of all epithelium-lined cysts of the jaws.

Epithelial debris from the dental lamina may be found in all parts of the jaws and, correspondingly, keratocysts may be found in almost any region. They are uncommon in the upper incisor region, but are seen fairly regularly in the upper molar, lower incisor and lower premolar regions. However, they are found most frequently in the ramus and lower third molar region. The reason for an undoubted propensity to involve this posterior site has not been explained satisfactorily. In the series reviewed by Shear at the Eastman Dental Hospital, London, there were 14 primordial cysts in the mandible and seven in the maxilla. The position of one cyst was unrecorded. Of the mandibular cysts, nine were sited in the lower third molar area, three in the premolar region and two extended throughout the entire body of the mandible. In the maxilla, three were identified in the third molar area, three in the vicinity of the premolars and one in the upper canine region. A study of 537 odontogenic cysts by Browne (1970) revealed an incidence of 7.6 per cent keratocysts, and the lesion was five times more common in the mandible than maxilla.

Clinical features

Primordial cysts may, on occasion, occur at a site where a tooth is absent from the adult dentition (Fig. 7.1). More commonly they start between the standing teeth, or distal to the last lower molar. They may extend around and between the teeth, or backwards into the ramus and up into the coronoid process, until they achieve a considerable size. Like other cysts in the mandible, expansion is delayed until the cortex is penetrated. In the maxilla, considerable enlargement into the maxillary sinus may occur before noticeable enlargement of the jaw takes place. Since there is not a pulpless tooth as in a radicular cyst, or an unerupted

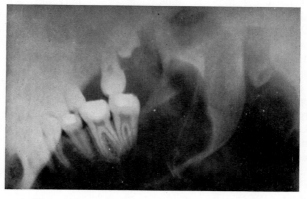

Fig. 7.1 Lateral oblique radiograph of an odontogenic keratocyst. Note that the /8 is absent.

tooth as seen in a dentigerous cyst, there may be little to attract the dental surgeon's clinical attention, so that a primordial cyst of the upper molar region may be mistaken for the maxillary sinus more readily than other types of cystic lesions. In advanced cases considerable expansion of the jaw occurs.

Odontogenic keratocysts usually remain symptomless until they become secondarily infected. Often the abnormality is discovered fortuitously on routine radiography. As has been mentioned, the extrafollicular dentigerous cyst does simulate a dentigerous cyst on clinical and radiographic examination. Parasthesia of the lower lip is unlikely unless the cyst becomes infected or unless a pathological fracture has occurred. The possibility of a malignant neoplasm having arisen in the lining should always be considered if mental anaesthesia is otherwise inexplicable.

In the tooth-bearing part of the jaw there may be more displacement of adjoining teeth than occurs with other cysts, because primordial cysts tend to extend to the buccal aspect of teeth in one part of the jaw and to the lingual in another, so displacing teeth in opposite directions (Figs. 7.2, 7.3). Age at identification of the lesion has ranged from 4 to 84 years (Sonesson 1950) but it is thought that they form early in life. A wide age distribution is confirmed by our own series, whereas Browne (1970) specified a peak incidence for diagnosis during the second and third decades.

Radiological examination (Figs. 7.4, 7.5)

Primordial cysts may be either unilocular or multilocular. The unilocular type is frequently indistinguishable from a radicular or a residual

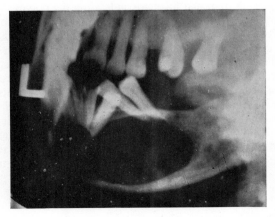

Fig. 7.2 Lateral oblique radiograph of a mandibular odontogenic keratocyst which has enlarged downwards and extended through the lower border of the jaw anteriorly. Note the deflection and resorption of tooth roots.

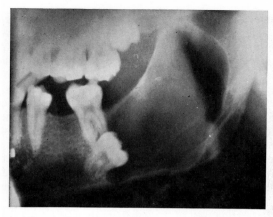

Fig. 7.3 Lateral oblique radiograph showing an odontogenic keratocyst which has displaced /8.

radicular cyst. Features which arouse suspicion are the presence of a cyst when all the teeth of the normal series are present and vital, or the occurrence of a cyst in a position such that its centre and presumed point of origin is distal to the dental arch. As with other unilocular cysts some may be in bony cavities with ridges on the walls which radiographically simulate bony septa.

Multilocular primordial cysts may have several radiographic appearances. Several cysts, usually one large one and several small ones, may be contained in one cavity in the bone, in which case there will be outpouchings of the bony cavity, some of which may have a circumference greater than half a sphere, indicating the polycystic nature of the contained lesion. In other cases, these outpouchings are so prominent that they give the cyst an amoeboid outline. Indeed, if serial films are available, a change in general shape may be noticeable with time. Such appearances are readily seen in the ramus and third molar region. It has been suggested (Seward 1963) that daughter cysts form and fuse with the primary cyst to give this appearance. Multiple, obvious, distinct bone cavities may be seen, some of which are superimposed partially upon one another. In some cases many cysts are present, forming a lesion which Bramley (1971) likened to a rabbit warren. Multilocular primordial cysts cannot be distinguished reliably from ameloblastoma on radiological grounds, and a biopsy is often necessary in such cases before treatment is undertaken.

Contents

Frequently the odontogenic keratocyst contains keratin, and at operation this is seen as inspissated, dirty-white material which has an

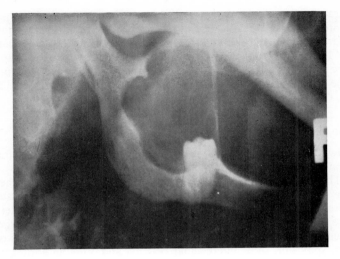

Fig. 7.4

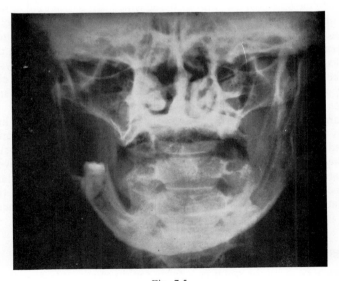

Fig. 7.5

Figs. 7.4 and 7.5 Radiographs of an odontogenic keratocyst in the angle and ramus of the mandible which has produced marked lingual expansion and cortical perforation.

appearance not unlike pus, but without an offensive smell. Aspiration is therefore a valuable diagnostic aid. A smear of the aspirate can be made, stained and examined for keratinized cells (Kramer 1970, Kramer and Toller 1973); electrophoresis may be undertaken, which will display a paucity of plasma proteins in the fluid (Toller 1967), or the total protein may be estimated and will be found to be below 4.0 g per 100 ml (Toller 1970).

Histological features

Browne (1971) generally supports Shear's criteria (p. 62) for the histopathological features of keratocysts. He states:

1. The lining is a regular continuous layer of stratified epithelium, usually six to eight cells thick, which arises from a smooth basement membrane. Frequently the epithelium is torn away from the underlying capsule. The basal cells are columnar, often exhibiting features suggestive of reversed polarity (in some cases they are cuboidal). The cells of the stratum spinosum show intercellular oedema and often an abrupt transition between them and the surface layer of keratin. The type of keratinization is that of parakeratosis. The keratinized surface is continuous over areas of focal inflammatory infiltrate.

2. The capsule is of thin fibrous tissue which is free from inflammatory cell infiltrate except for occasional focal accumulations. Cholesterol clefts are uncommon. Infection, particularly chronic infection, can alter the appearance so much that the lining is less easy to distinguish from that of a radicular cyst. Even so, Browne (1971) feels that parts of the cyst wall are likely to exhibit the characteristic features. Tiny patches of ciliated and mucus-secreting cells may also be found, but their extent and incidence is much lower than that in other cysts of the jaws.

Main (1970b) determined the mitotic value for various cyst linings. This is the number of mitoses per unit length of basement membrane. He showed a level of mitotic activity about twice that of radicular cysts and even higher proportionately than that of other simple cysts. The level was comparable with that found in ameloblastoma and dental lamina. Browne (1971) found a mitotic rate of 0.74 per 1500 cells. From this he calculated a mitotic value of about 3.9 which is similar to that found by Main for radicular cysts.

Enlargement of keratocysts

Clinical observation suggests a fairly rapid growth, at least in the early stages, for cysts may recur while the patient is under postoperative follow-up. Whether large keratocysts also enlarge rapidly is not known, because of the few symptoms associated with their presence and the lack of indication of the possible time of onset. By contrast, some small keratocysts are known to remain the same size over some years.

Whether this speed of enlargement of recurrent cysts is related to the mitotic activity of the epithelium is a subject for speculation. It has been suggested that the lobulated periphery of some examples is due to the pultaceous or semi-solid nature of the contents (Kramer 1974). It is postulated that if fresh desquamated cells were added at certain parts more rapidly than at others, they would result in localized pressure resorption. However, the mass inside the cyst is never dry and never more than semi-solid. Particulate matter which has all the interstices filled with liquid behaves like a liquid (as, for example, in the case of quicksand) and consequently the internal pressure remains distributed equally.

Recurrence of keratocysts (Figs. 7.6–7.9)

The tendency for keratocysts to recur was mentioned by Catania (1952). Seward (1962) gave the percentage recurrence in his experience as 40 per cent. Pindborg and Hansen (1963) and Toller (1967) suggested it might be as high as 60 per cent. Killey and Kay (1972) found the incidence lower. Browne (1970) advocated a follow-up period of a minimum of five years.

Most surgeons recognize that many cysts which recur may do so repeatedly. This means that the incidence of patients with recurring keratocysts is lower than the incidence of recurrent cysts. Further, not all new cysts in patients with the multiple cyst syndrome are recurrences.

The possible reasons for recurrence are many. Frequently the cyst lining is thin and delicate, and at operation fragments of lining may be retained. Cysts frequently penetrate the original cortex of the jaw and, also, eventually, the thin shell of subperiosteal new bone. With the relatively tough membrane of other cyst linings it is not too difficult, with patience and reasonable access, to separate the lining from the resilient mucoperiosteum of nose, antrum or palate. It is much more difficult to separate a cyst lining from periosteum and overlying muscle, as in the ramus region of the mandible, the lingual side of the molar alveolar process and the posterior aspect of the maxilla. With the fragile lining of a keratocyst, attempts to elevate the periosteum from the surface of the lesion usually result in perforation of the cyst sac and the spilling of cyst contents. Attempts to strip the lining from the periosteum working from within the bony cavity frequently end with a tear in the lining. From this point on the chance that a fragment of lining may be left behind is considerable. Recurrence therefore may follow the retention of fragments of lining, or possibly from the seeding of viable epithelial cells into the tissues. Where the tissue planes have been more widely opened, as when a submandibular approach is made to the mandible, recurrence may result in the soft tissues (Emerson *et al.* 1972).

Browne (1971) distinguishes between satellite cysts found in the cyst capsule and epithelial residues, presumably of dental lamina. He agrees

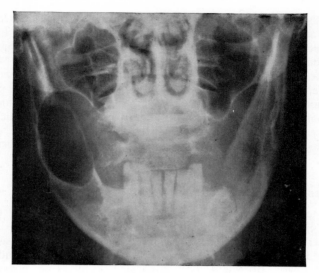

Fig. 7.6

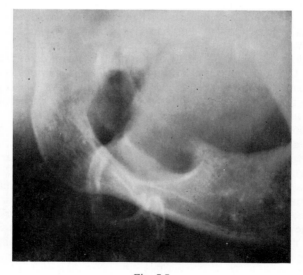

Fig. 7.7

Figs. 7.6 and 7.7 Postero-anterior and lateral oblique radiographs of an odontogenic keratocyst in the ramus of the mandible.

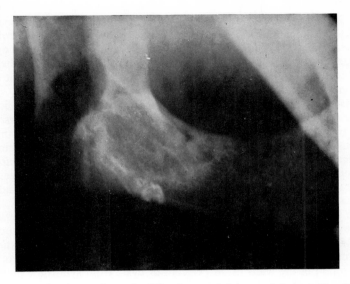

Fig. 7.8 Lateral oblique radiograph of the odontogenic keratocyst shown in Figs. 7.6 and 7.7 two years after operation showing obliteration of the bone cavity with new bone.

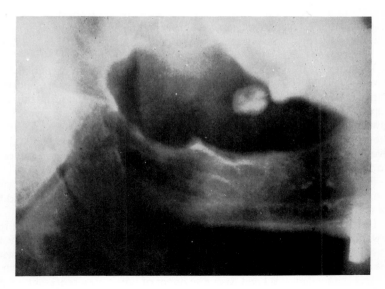

Fig. 7.9 Lateral oblique radiograph of the odontogenic keratocyst shown in Figs. 7.6 and 7.7 showing recurrence four years after operation.

with Soskolne and Shear (1967) that the satellite cysts probably arise from the epithelial residues rather than the outgrowth of cells from the basal layers of the main cyst. He therefore takes the view that the cystic change is multicentric. On the other hand, proliferations of epithelium from the basal layers of cysts into the capsule can be found, and it may be a matter of chance whether sections show a connection.

It is the experience of most operators that cysts in an extrafollicular dentigerous relationship are less likely to recur than primordial cysts. It is also true that they more often occupy a single bony compartment, although daughter cysts, perhaps of some size, may be found within the enucleated specimen. Browne (1971) contends that cysts *without* epithelial remnants in the capsule are more likely to recur. The suggestion is that the potentially active epithelium is in the adjacent medullary spaces.

On the other hand, Payne (1972) reports that a bud-like proliferation of the basal layer was observed in 45 per cent of recurrent keratocysts and 45 per cent of keratocysts from basal-cell naevus syndrome patients, but in only 8 per cent of non-recurrent keratocysts. Similarly, microcysts were found in the walls of 78 per cent of cysts from syndrome patients, 18 per cent of recurrent keratocysts and 4 per cent of non-recurrent cysts.

It is also noted by Browne (1971) that some of the microscopic satellite cysts undergo degeneration and end as a mass of keratin which is removed by giant cells. Similar changes are seen in some gingival and periodontal cysts which may well be a form of keratocyst. Thus, to a degree, there is a contradiction in the behaviour of these cysts. On the one hand there is a strong tendency to recur, and on the other, evidence of spontaneous degeneration of some satellite cysts.

Recurrence, therefore, may follow the failure to remove potentially active epithelial residues. If the view is taken that all of these represent remnants of the original dental lamina, then the residues found in the cyst capsule are of no more (or less) significance than those in the rest of the jaw. There is some evidence, in the form of proliferation outwards from the epithelium lining the cyst, that some may be newly formed and of active epithelial cells. The removal of these epithelial cells is clearly important.

Recurrence may also follow the retention of satellite cysts. Such cysts may be discovered at times in specimens of medullary bone removed to gain access to the cyst cavity.

In some cases the new cysts arise in previously uninvolved parts of the jaw. Such occurrences may be indicative of a widespread tendency to cyst formation affecting the residues of the dental lamina. Patients with the basal-cell naevus–multiple cyst syndrome have such a propensity. Where the tendency is local to one segment of jaw it may represent a field change. Strictly speaking, even recurrence due to the retention of a satellite cyst is only separated from such a process by a matter of degree.

An interesting concept of the occurrence and recurrence of keratocysts stems from observations by Braden *et al.* (1968), Stoelinga (1973) and Stoelinga and Peters (1973). Braden *et al.* described two small nodular lesions from the canine–premolar region and an ulcerated lesion from a similar location. These lesions contained a multitude of rests and strands of odontogenic epithelium, some of which appeared to be in direct continuity with the basal layers of the oral mucosa. These exhibited the so-called 'dropping-off' phenomenon. Braden *et al.* described these nodules as hamartomas of the dental lamina. Somewhat similar lesions have been described in relation to gingival cysts.

The frequent occurrence of epithelial rests at and distal to the lower third molar region is generally recognized. Stoelinga and Peters (1973) investigated the growth backwards of the dental lamina in human and monkey material. They noted that the mucosa overlying keratocysts was adherent to the cyst lining through fenestrations in the bone. They excised the mucosa with the lining and demonstrated that epithelial islands and daughter cysts were present only in the mucosa. They advocate the excision of the overlying mucosa as a means of preventing recurrence. Harris (1974) feels that a trial of this method is worth while. Certainly, in some cases of primordial cyst of the ramus, there is a channel through the bone backwards from the alveolar crest in the third molar region, similar to that seen leading to a young third molar tooth germ. Some keratocysts occurring more anteriorly in the jaws may also be connected to the overlying mucosa by a strand of fibrous tissue, which passes through an opening in the bone like a gubernacular canal. On the other hand many recurrences occur deep in the jaw and remote from the overlying mucosa.

Treatment

An attempt to suggest logical case management was made by Bramley (1971). He emphasized that treatment must be based on an accurate diagnosis, and that appropriate tests should be carried out on an aspirate of the cyst contents to this end. Unilocular cysts he suggests should be enucleated by an intraoral approach. Where access is difficult, primary decompression is followed by secondary enucleation at a later date.

For those cysts with a loculated periphery but a single bone cavity he advocates resection of the containing block of bone, short of complete section of the jaw wherever this is possible. Otherwise careful enucleation is performed, with regular follow-up to detect any recurrence.

Multilocular cysts which honeycomb the jaw should be treated by excision of the containing block of bone. Often this means resection of a sizeable length of jaw and immediate bone graft.

In the authors' experience it has been found possible to treat both of the first two types by enucleation. Either type may recur, but if careful follow-up is pursued the new cyst will be small and again be enucleated. Sometimes this process must be repeated several times, but if care is taken to operate through the mouth and to avoid the opening up of tissue planes no harm results, and eventually further recurrence will not take place. The process of marsupialization and secondary enucleation would seem to be illogical, as regeneration of bone takes place by penetration of the capsule by new bone trabeculae. There would seem to be every likelihood of the incorporation of epithelial rests within the new bone. Nevertheless there are occasional indications for this method. One indication for this technique is where it is wished to conserve anterior teeth in a child and the roots have been denuded, perhaps by an extrafollicular dentigerous cyst. Bramley's approach to the highly multilocular cyst is the only practical method. In such a case it is important firstly to section the jaw beyond the involved portion, and secondly to divide the soft tissue with knife or scissors a short distance away from any perforations of the bone. Unless this is done, the cysts will still be torn and recurrence in the soft tissues or bone graft may follow.

REFERENCES

Braden, E., Moskow, B. S. & Moskow, R. (1968) *J. oral Surg.,* **26,** 702.
Bernier, J. L. (1955) *The Management of Oral Disease.* St. Louis Mosby.
Bramley, P. A. (1971) *Proc. Roy. Soc. Med.,* **64,** 547.
Browne, R. M. (1970) *Brit. dent. J.,* **128,** 225.
Browne, R. M. (1971) *Brit. dent. J.,* **131,** 249.
Catania, A. F. (1952) *Oral. Surg.,* **5,** 895.
Emerson, T. G., Whitlock, R. I. H. & Jones, J. H. (1972) *Brit. J. Oral Surg.,* **9,** 181.
Harris, M. (1974) *Prostaglandin production and bone resorption by dental cysts.* Hunterian Lecture at the Royal College of Surgeons of England, 15 March 1974.
Harris, M. (1974) *Proc. Roy. Soc. Med.,* **67,** 1259.
Killey, H. C., & Kay, L. W. (1972) *Benign Cystic Lesions of the Jaws, their Diagnosis and Treatment,* 2nd ed. Edinburgh: Churchill Livingstone.
Kramer, I. R. H. (1970) Letter to the editor, *Brit. dent. J.,* **128,** 370.
Kramer, I. R. H., & Toller, P. A. (1973) *Int. J. Oral Surg.,* **2,** 143.
Kramer, I. R. H. (1974) *Proc. Roy. Soc. Med.,* **67,** 27'.
Magitot, E. (1872) *Arch. Gèn. Med.,* **2,** 399–414, 681.
Main, D. M. G., (1970a) *Odontological Revy,* **21,** 29.
Main, D. M. G. (1970b) *Brit. J. Oral Surg.,* **8,** 114.
Payne, T. F. (1972) *Oral Surg.,* **33,** 538.
Philipsen, H. P. (1956) *Tandlaegebladet,* **60,** 963.
Pindborg, J. J. & Hansen, J. (1963) *Acta path. microbiol. scand.,* **58,** 283.
Robinson, H. B. G. (1945) *A. J. Orthodont. Oral Surg.* (Oral Surg. Sec.), **31,** 370.
Seward, G. R. (1962) Paper presented at BDA Annual Conference, Nottingham, 18 July 1962.
Seward, G. R. (1963) *Brit. dent. J.,* **115,** 231.
Shafer, W. G., Hine, M. K., & Levy, B. M. (1963) *A Textbook of Oral Pathology.* Philadelphia: Saunders.
Shear, M. (1960) *Jour. D.A.S.A.,* **15,** 211.
Sonesson, A. (1950) *Acta Radiol.* Suppl. 81.
Soskolne, W. A. & Shear, M. (1967) *Brit. dent. J.,* **123,** 321.
Stoelinga, P. J. W. (1973) In Kay, L. W. (ed.), *Oral Surgery,* p. 77: Churchill Livingstone. Edinburgh.
Stoelinga, P. J. W. & Peters, J. H. (1973) *Int. J. Oral Surg.* **2,** 37.
Toller, P. A. (1967) *Ann. Roy. Coll. Surg.,* **40,** 306.
Toller, P. A. (1970) *Brit. dent J.,* **128,** 317.

8. Non-Keratinizing Cysts

Eruption cysts

As has been seen, eruption cysts are superficial cysts similar in their relationship to the crown of the tooth as the dentigerous cyst. They are most commonly seen over erupting primary molars (Seward 1973) and present as a tense, dark blue or purple swelling. Spontaneous rupture followed by eruption of the tooth is usual. Very occasionally this does not happen and the child is occasioned much pain. If the episode is unreasonably prolonged, simple incision of the cyst is followed by relief of symptoms and eruption of the tooth.

Eruption cysts may be seen occasionally over first molars or even premolars where the primary tooth has been extracted some time before. They do not occasion destruction of bone and do not result in a bony cavity. Such cysts must be distinguished from dentigerous cysts which have enlarged to present at the alveolar crest as a bluish swelling. They are lined by a thin layer of stratified squamous epithelium, but may show sizeable epithelial discontinuities. Their origin is discussed with that of dentigerous cysts (p. 94).

Radicular cysts

Periapical radicular cysts

Of all cystic lesions in the jaws this is the most common. In all cases the pulp of the related tooth has become necrosed. Whether in all cases the root canal is infected, or whether cysts can develop in response to the presence of a sterile but necrotic pulp, is not known. In the majority of cases the tooth dies from an extension of gross caries, but alternative causes are fractures of the tooth which expose the pulp, pulpal exposures during cavity preparation and the ingress of organisms through the imperfect enamel and dentine within a cingulum invagination or dens in dente. Pulps may undergo sterile necrosis as the result of an acute, closed pulpitis incited by the heat of incautious cavity preparation, a chemically irritant filling material, or by trauma which damages the apical blood supply. Infection frequently reaches the necrotic tissues indirectly, but as was stated above, it is not known if this is essential for the development of a cyst. The work of Seltzer et al. (1969), which involved stimulation of the periapical tissues with sterile instruments or sterile root filling materials, suggests that infection is not essential, in that typical epithelial rest proliferation occurred in these experiments.

The initiation of radicular cysts

Following bacterial invasion of the pulp, micro-organisms reach the periapical tissues and a chronic low-grade infection leads to the formation of a periapical granuloma. Around a healthy tooth the epithelial cell rests of Malassez form a network in the periodontal membrane. These cells are normally metabolically quiescent. They each have a dark nucleus and a narrow rim of cytoplasm (Ten Cate 1972). With the formation of a granuloma the adjacent epithelial cells are activated and proliferate. In histological preparations their nuclei are paler and there is a marked increase in the amounts of cytoplasm. Valderhaug (1972) has shown that the epithelium proliferates to form strands, arcades and rings at the junction of the uninflamed connective tissue and the granulation tissue. Malassez (1887) was the first to suggest that apical cysts originated from these proliferating epithelial remnants.

The formation of a cavity lined by epithelium could occur by a number of mechanisms. For instance, epithelial cells will proliferate to cover a connective tissue surface. If clefts produced by the accumulation of a purulent exudate in the form of microabscesses involved one of the proliferating strands of epithelium, the epithelial cells would be expected to line the cleft. Indeed, Powell White (1910) showed that if sterile abscesses which resulted from the injection of oleic acid subdermally came into contact with epidermal structures such as hair follicle, they would become lined with epithelium. Ledingham (1933) produced subcutaneous abscesses in guinea-pigs which became lined with epithelium in a similar fashion.

At one time it was thought – as an alternative mechanism – that the epithelium proliferated to form a sphere of cells. Death of the central cells was postulated on the grounds that the mass would grow so large that diffusion of oxygen and nutrients would be insufficient to maintain them. In fact, masses of cells of a size to make this mechanism likely are not seen. However, epithelial cells become orientated in relation to their source of nutrition and the adjacent connective tissue. When in the normal situation they cover a surface and are finally desquamated. If the proliferating epithelium is beneath the surface as in a granuloma, the cells will migrate inwards and will desquamate in the centre of the mass. Such a progression is seen in the epithelial pearls and microcysts in the midline of the palate of neonates, and in epithelial pearls in squamous cell epitheliomas. This is the probable mechanism by which inclusion cysts such as sublingual dermoids are formed. Ten Cate (1972) has demonstrated death of the central cells of the proliferating strands of epithelium in experimentally induced periapical granulomas in monkeys.

Harris (1974) suggests that the spongework of epithelial cells at the periphery of a granuloma plays a protective role, isolating the irritating and infected material in the centre. Valderhaug (1972) and Harris (1974) also suggest that the entire centre of the granuloma becomes necrotic, and that following this the cell meshwork becomes consolidated into the familiar epithelium-lined cyst sac. Shear (1963) likewise observes that the early developing periodontal cyst is surrounded by proliferating arcades and rings of epithelium, each with a vascular connective tissue core and that later this arcade pattern disappears.

Enlargement of radicular cysts

It may be that the mechanism governing enlargement of cysts of the jaw is the same, irrespective of the type of cyst. Alternatively a different mechanism may be involved for each of the different types or various groups of cysts. Another possibility is that the basic mechanism is similar, but there are additional factors involved which differ from type to type. The latter possibility seems the most likely. The various factors which are involved seem to be as follows:

1. The production of a raised internal hydrostatic pressure.
2. The attraction of fluid into the cyst cavity.
3. The retention of the fluid within the cavity.
4. The resorption of the surrounding bone with an increase in the size of the bony cavity.

In his Hunterian Lecture, Harris (1974) classified the theories of cyst enlargement in the following manner:

1. Mural growth
   (a) Peripheral cell division
   (b) Accumulated contents
2. Hydrostatic
   (a) Secretion
   (b) Transudation and exudation
   (c) Dialysis

This classification is similar to that used by Main (1970).

The mural growth mechanisms are discussed in the chapter on keratocysts (p. 62).

The creation of an increased intraluminal pressure by secretion is unlikely normally to be a factor, since only occasionally are mucus-secreting goblet cells to be found in the lining of radicular cysts.

1. *The raised internal hydrostatic pressure.* In 1926, Warwick James attempted to measure the intraluminal pressure of several uninfected cysts in vivo. He introduced a cannula into the cysts and connected it to a mercury or aneroid manometer. He recorded pressures of 12 to 100 centimetres of water.

Later in 1948 Toller confirmed these results, using the more sensitive water manometer. He found pressures averaging 70 centimetres of water (range 56.6 to 95.0 cmH_2O) in 51 radicular cysts, 65 centimetres of water (range 22.5 to 94.7 cmH_2O) in 9 dentigerous cysts and 87.5 centimetres of water in an anterior developmental cyst.

It has been suggested (Harris 1974) that what is measured by a manometer inserted into a cyst lumen is the elasticity in the wall and the vascular pressure of the cyst capsule. The latter is, of course, exerted between the wall of the bony cavity and the liquid contents of the cyst, and hence transmitted to the manometer when the cavity is opened to the manometric system. Presumably as the cavity is decompressed there could be an increase in volume of the vascular bed. This would increase the amount of fluid displaced into the manometer.

The amount of elasticity exhibited by a cyst sac which is still adherent to the bony wall of the cyst cavity is unknown – as, indeed, is the elasticity of the isolated cyst sac. Such elasticity would be ·due only to the collagen fibres in the capsule as there are no elastic fibres in the capsule.

2. *The attraction of fluid into the cyst cavity.* Dialysis, as a result of the higher osmolarity of cyst fluid than serum, is the most commonly favoured mechanism. Warwick James (1926), Tratman (1939), Sealey (1948), Toller (1948 and 1970) and Stokke (1956) have all produced evidence which supports this point of view.

First Stokke in 1956 and then Toller in 1970 measured the vapour pressure of cyst fluids. Osmotic pressure is related to the number of dissolved particles in a solution. Osmolarity is the number of these dissolved particles. Since vapour pressure is also related to the number of particles dispersed in a solution, a measure of vapour pressure can be used as an indirect means of measuring osmolarity. Toller records that in 34 cases out of 44 the osmolarity of the cyst fluids was higher than that of the patients' own serum. In 3 cases the serum and the fluid were isotonic, and in 4 out of the 7 cases in which the serum osmolarity was the higher the difference was less than the experimental error of the method. In 15 cases the osmotic difference was compared with a measurement of the total soluble protein in the cyst fluids; no such correlation was established. This was taken as supporting the concept that the raised osmolarity was due to the liberation of products of cellular lysis, which may not be proteins.

The most commonly accepted mechanism is a simple one, namely that desquamated epithelial cells of the cyst lining undergo autolysis and so produce a larger number of molecules of lower molecular weight, thus raising the osmolarity of the fluid. Water from tissue fluid in the surrounding tissues is attracted into the cyst so raising its internal pressure. This hydrostatic force is ultimately transmitted to the adjacent bone so inducing pressure resorption. The state of osmotic imbalance is maintained by the constant turnover of epithelial cells which are then shed into the cyst space. Harris (1974) sees certain difficulties in this simple explanation. The cyst fluids contain albumin which does not normally cross physiological semipermeable membranes in any quantity. He has also shown the presence of much larger molecules such as fibrin and its breakdown products which could only reach the cyst lumen through highly permeable capillary walls such as are found in inflamed tissue.

Main (1970) has reviewed other mechanisms whereby cyst fluid may accumulate inside the cyst cavity and if possible accumulate in such a way as to create a raised intraluminal pressure. He too discounts secretion and feels that osmosis cannot be entirely endorsed. He considers exudation of a protein-rich fluid through capillaries made more permeable by acute inflammation. Whilst any cyst may become acutely infected and inflamed, this is not the normal and continuing state of affairs. Indeed, marked hyperemia is commonly a feature only of the very early radicular cyst, before the typical, even lining epithelium has been established. A chronic inflammatory cell infiltrate is seen in radicular cyst walls, and with it, presumably, appropriate vascular changes, but it is absent from all other cyst linings unless secondary infection has occurred. In a limited experiment, reported in the same paper, in which the specific gravity of cyst fluids was determined, results suggestive of an exudate were obtained from radicular cysts with acute inflammatory changes superimposed on those of chronic inflammation of the lining and a transudative type of specific gravity from an inflamed lining which had perforated the cortical plate. A transudative type of measurement was also obtained from two dentigerous cysts.

Main (1970) also discusses transudation as a result of venous obstruction. He points out that if a cyst has a high internal hydrostatic pressure the venous pressure might exceed 55 centimetres of water, at which level endothelial permeability would be markedly altered so as to allow considerable additional protein leakage (Walter and Israel 1963). Such a mechanism, namely the compression of the cyst lining to a degree which would produce some increase in venous pressure (but without arresting the circulation), might account for a protein content of the cyst fluid which otherwise might be difficult to explain.

3. *Retention of fluid within the cyst cavity.* If the osmolic–dialysis concept is accepted, fluid is attracted into the cyst cavity by the products of epithelial cell autolysis which by themselves are unable to diffuse out of the cavity. Toller (1966) noted that albumin was present in amounts similar to plasma in radicular and dentigerous cysts, but there were very small amounts of the proteins with a larger molecular size. In keratocysts only a slight amount of soluble protein entered the cyst. Thus, there was a selective admission of molecules into the cyst. If this dialysis was through a simple semipermeable membrane it would be expected that molecules could escape from the cyst through the membrane in the same way. Since albumin would be likely to be a molecule of larger size than the products of epithelial cell autolysis, these products should be able to diffuse out and thus would not create the postulated osmotic imbalance.

In further experiments (Toller 1967) Toller introduced radioactive labelled crystalloid (^{24}NaCl) and human albumin tagged with ^{131}I, both suspended in isotonic saline, into cysts from which the cyst fluid had been evacuated. The crystalloid diffused out of the cyst fairly rapidly during the first twenty-four hours, but the albumin was largely retained and escaped much more slowly. In other experiments (Toller 1966) a dye of large molecular weight (Patent blue) was instilled as an 11 per cent sterile isotonic aqueous solution into seven cysts which had been aspirated to remove the original cyst fluid. At operation it was found that the dye remained confined to the cavity, in spite of the fact that this material is normally injected in order that it may be taken up into the lymphatics so that the latter can be identified in lymphangiography. Toller, therefore, postulated that the osmotic imbalance resulted from the inability of the larger molecules to escape because of the lack of access to the lymphatic system. Thus, there is a semipermeable membrane mechanism governing access into the cyst, and a lack of lymphatic access acting as a bar to the escape of certain substances from their contents. By this mechanism, it seems more likely that the products of epithelial autolysis could effect the osmotic attraction and retention of fluid within cyst cavities.

4. *Resorption of bone and enlargement of the cyst.* The generally accepted mechanism for the enlargement of cysts of the jaws is that the positive internal pressure is transmitted to the adjacent bone which undergoes resorption. In this way, the bony cavity is enlarged, permitting further fluid – attracted into the lumen of the cyst – to increase its volume and re-establish the internal pressure. As a consequence of these changes the surface area of the cyst lining is increased by cell multiplication. As a result of an induction effect of the epithelial cells a connective tissue capsule is formed between the epithelium and the bone (Harris 1974).

The objection is raised that the expansile force of the cyst fluid might be counterbalanced by a contractile force of the cyst capsule, or at least by the creation of a tension within a capsule of limited extensibility. A counterbalancing force due to the ability of the cyst lining to contain and resist the expansile pressure of the fluid, so reaching an equilibrium, is easy to understand for a cyst surrounded by unresistant soft tissues. Enlargement would occur due to growth in an area of the cyst lining and, by attraction of fluid into the interior, so increasing its volume and maintaining the internal pressure. But, like a balloon, the tension in the wall would balance the internal pressure. Thus, there would be no positive pressure against the surrounding tissues which would simply be displaced.

Where the cyst sac is itself enclosed in a bony compartment which it fills completely, another set of circumstances exists, particularly as the cyst sac is adherent to the bony wall, and it would seem possible for pressure to be transmitted to the inside of the bony cavity. The limiting factor would be the circulation of blood within the vessels of the cyst capsule. If the pressure were sufficient to compress the blood vessels the capsule would necrose. The situation is analogous to successful orthodontic movement of a tooth. Here, the pressure is transmitted to the bone from the tooth root via the periodontal membrane, but must not be sufficient to impair the circulation. The process is, of course, a dynamic one for if the increments of pressure occurred slowly and bone resorption took place in response to the pressure, the critical degree of pressure for bone resorption might be maintained without an adverse effect upon the capsular circulation. However, should the venous side of the capsular vasculature be impeded to some degree this could account for the passage of certain plasma proteins into the cyst fluid. The actual proteins reaching the fluid depend in part on the permeability of the lining — i.e., whether there is an epithelial layer, whether the epithelium is discontinuous or whether it is keratinized or unkeratinized.

Recently Harris and Goldhaber (1973) have shown that living explants of cyst lining induce rapid resorption of the bone of a mouse calvarium. Harris *et al.* (1973) have produced evidence that components of the bone resorbing factor are the prostaglandins PGE_2 and possibly PGE_3 or PGF_3. The ability of these explants of cyst lining to induce the resorption of bone is certainly striking. The means by which such a mechanism might be activated and inactivated *in vivo* remains to be determined.

Certainly the removal of fluid from within a cyst, either by repeated aspiration or drainage via an incision or an open root canal is sufficient to reverse the process of enlargement and permit new bone to be laid down in the capsule. The time-honoured methods of treatment by the insertion of a self-retaining grommet in a hole in the cyst wall, or by marsupialization, also appears to depend upon decompressing the cyst. In these cases, the cyst lining is still in contact with bone, suggesting that either pressure or the presence of cyst fluid within the cyst may be required for activation of the prostaglandin mechanism. However, since neither of these factors seem to be involved in the mouse calvarium experiments, perhaps some other trigger mechanism may be responsible.

The rate of enlargement of radicular cysts

An estimate was made by Livingstone (1927) of the annual increase in growth of a periodontal cyst which specified an enlargement in diameter of approximately 5 mm per year. During a survey of 500 cysts of the jaws, one of the authors was responsible in some instances for recording cyst size in relationship to the time since the death of the tooth pulp. This was judged in some cases by the stage at which tooth development was arrested in incompletely formed teeth. In other cases, the time at which the pulp irritating stimulus was applied was known. These observations suggested that in teenaged patients and adults, about ten years is required for the development of a cyst 2 cm in diameter. There is evidence that in younger subjects much more rapid cyst enlargement is possible. Shear (1963) suggests that the larger the cyst the slower the yearly increase in diameter. The diameter of 2 cm is a critical size beyond which it is likely that expansion of the jaw will be detected clinically.

Relatively, the incidence of periodontal cysts is highest in the maxilla, and in this jaw they are most frequently located anteriorly. In contradistinction, mandibular cysts mainly arise in the posterior region. Individually the tooth most commonly incriminated in this type of cyst formation is the maxillary second incisor. This small tooth has a pulp chamber in close proximity to the external surface; it is prone to caries, to inadvertent trauma because of its position and is liable to insidious pulpal death as a result of a developmental defect or from insufficient pulpal protection against the toxic or irritant effects of synthetic restorative materials.

Sex difference in the incidence of periodontal cysts is not appreciable, but males tend to be affected more than females, presumably because the latter are more conscious of their appearance and seek dental attention more assiduously. Apical cysts may be associated with teeth both in the primary and secondary dentitions, but occurrence is uncommon in the deciduous series and unusual even in adolescence. In the adult, the common age of occurrence is in the fourth decade. Despite its slow growth the cyst may attain large proportions and involve a whole quadrant before the diagnosis is made.

The pressure exerted by a cyst has been likened by Cowan (1953) to that of a balloon filled with air in a confined space – the force is equal in all directions and so, potentially, expansion is symmetrical. Perhaps a water-filled balloon is a closer analogy. Nevertheless, in a uniform environment the cyst would be spherical in shape, but contact with structures offering varying degrees of resistance causes a differential bone resorption and consequent modification to the cyst outline. The resistance to lateral enlargement offered by the thick cortex of the mandible leads to involvement of much of the medullary cavity in some cases before clinical diagnosis is possible. Conversely, in the maxilla the air-filled maxillary sinuses and the inferior meatus of the nose are exploited before enlargement into the sulcus or palate occurs, and again a complaint by the patient tends to be delayed.

There is an inclination to regard radicular cysts as solitary lesions related to indvidual teeth, yet it is not exceptional to discover two, three or more concurrent cysts on the apices of carious teeth or roots in different parts of the mouth. Indeed, there may be a separate small cyst arising from each apex of a multi-rooted tooth. Some of these discrete, small cysts may merge after prolonged growth due to destruction of their intervening walls. In the course of this transition to a monolocular cavity, it is obvious that an incidental radiograph of the jaw taken at this period would reveal a loculated lesion.

Clinical findings

Discovery of a cyst is often made by chance as a result of routine radiography, for a considerable period of time may elapse before the lesion is apparent clinically. Few cysts smaller than 2 cm in diameter produce a readily detectable swelling. Indeed symptoms may remain insignificant until suppuration is superimposed with resultant pain. The various consistencies of an enlargement, which vary according to the thickness of the overlying bone, have been described previously. At the final stage, when bone destruction outstrips subperiosteal new bone formation, frank fluctuation of the smooth-surfaced swelling will be confirmed. In the mandible, labial or buccal expansion occurs predominantly, and lingual protrusion tends to be seen more in the third molar region and ramus. However, expansion in the premolar or first molar region may occur and may be overlooked, either because it is below the level of the floor of the mouth and not felt for specifically, or because the occlusal films are taken with the beam tangential to the buccal rather than the lingual cortex.

Some periapical cysts of the maxilla may bulge outwards initially, but not those associated with the posteriorly inclined root of the lateral incisor and the palatal roots of the first premolar and upper molars. From these teeth cysts may be found which expand only the palate. The mucosa overlying the cystic expansion, which is at first of normal colour, may then become conspicuous because of the dilated blood vessels, and finally take on a profound dark blue tinge.

An associated intraoral sinus discharging pus or brownish fluid may form after the cyst becomes infected, and occasionally a chronic sinus track may be established which leads externally to the face or neck. Confirmation of the vitality of the pulps of all teeth related to a cystic lesion would rule out a diagnosis of apical cyst, except for the unlikely possibility of a cyst forming after pulpal infection of a single root of a molar tooth whose remaining root canals are healthy. The pulpless tooth responsible for the cyst may be slightly loose or have an evident carious exposure, or merely a dark discoloration when death of the tooth has followed a traumatic injury. Occasionally the affected tooth is sensitive to percussion.

Teeth bordering upon the cystic lesion may be slightly mobile, although this is uncommon. Where the cyst is large they may be displaced. Instances of a temporary pressure neuritis of the peripheral sensory nerve to either the upper or lower lip are not unusual following suppuration in a cyst. The hallmark will be anaesthesia or paraesthesia over the area of distribution. Pathological fracture through a large cyst cavity is another possible mode of presentation.

Radiological examination

The small or moderate-sized apical periodontal cyst appears as a spheroidal, pear or flask-shaped area of radiolucency enclosed by a distinct margin which merges with the lamina dura of the causative tooth. However, apical to the point of junction of cyst rim to tooth, the lamina dura is deficient. According to Ingram (1965) the condensed peripheral line is better developed with slow-growing cysts which occur in the older patient. In contrast he stresses that periodontal cysts in young jaws have a discrete margin, but often lack a line of compact bone. Sonesson (1950) pointed out that contrary to popular opinion only a small percentage of radiographs of cysts show a white line at the bone cavity. Critical inspec-

D

tion of radiographs will reveal the following state of affairs. In the case of about one-third of large granulomas or small cysts there is a thin radio-opaque margin to the bone cavity. In the case of larger cysts rather fewer examples have a white peripheral line where the cavity margin is formed by cancellous bone. However, over the expanded part of the jaw, a sheet of subperiosteal new bone is laid down and this will produce a white linear image. In some cases this line will be superimposed by chance over part of the periphery within the jaw. In other cases an appearance resembling a septum will be produced. Rotation of the jaw or attenuation of the angle of the X-ray beam will either move the line away from the periphery or cause the beam to pass obliquely to the sheet of bone and no longer cast a linear image (Seward 1963).

Root apices of teeth encompassed by the cyst may undergo a shallow, even resorption due to pressure (Figs. 8.1–8.3). But often they remain vital, and when the tension has been relieved by treatment the lamina dura will re-form around the truncated root ends. The trabeculae of the surrounding bone are invariably normal.

Impediment to expansion leads to eccentric growth and therefore to irregular shapes, and a large cyst may lose definition of outline. The effect of superimposed infection upon the cyst circumference has been detailed previously.

There is a close resemblance between the radiographic appearance of a chronic periapical abscess or granuloma and that of a small apical cyst, which may lead to difficulty in differentiation. Despite the similarity, agreement on an arbitrary means of distinction has been reached: if the apical area at the apex of a non-vital tooth is over 1 cm in diameter it is very likely to be a cyst and not a granuloma. The periapical radiolucency of a cementoma in its earliest stage may be erroneously diagnosed as an apical cyst but the important point of dissimilarity is the vitality of the associated tooth. In the radiographic image of a periodontal cyst it is sometimes possible to discern calcification in the cyst wall, which Rushton and Cooke (1959) compared with the metastatic calcification found in degenerating epithelial cells and fibrous tissue that had been the site of chronic inflammation elsewhere in the body. These calcifications are not to be confused with those occurring in the lining of the calcifying odontogenic cyst and in the adenoameloblastoma.

Contents

The cyst fluid is straw-coloured and glairy with an iridescent sheen imparted by the cholesterol crystal content. The protein concentration is between 5.0 and 11.0 g per 100 ml with a mean level of the same order as blood serum (Toller 1970), and a small amount of keratin material may be identified. When infection supervenes the cyst may contain pus, seropurulent or sanguinopurulent fluid, but from time to time on opening a cyst sac, material of paste-like or caseous consistency can be expressed. On microscopic section polymorphonuclear leucocytes, foam cells and cholesterol clefts may be seen.

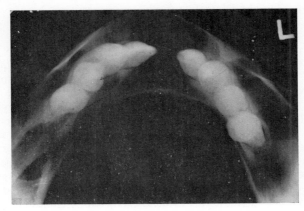

Fig. 8.1

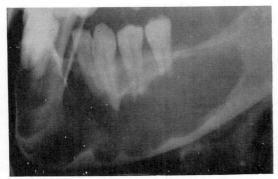

Fig. 8.2

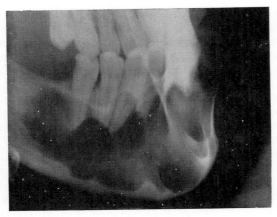

Fig. 8.3

Figs. 8.1 to 8.3 Lateral oblique and occlusal radiographs of a periodontal cyst with a lobulated periphery occupying the greater part of the body of the mandible. The roots of the majority of the involved teeth were eroded, and these were removed together with the cyst lining. A primary closure was performed.

Pathological examination

Young cysts are lined by a thick hyperplastic stratified squamous epithelium. Microcysts form sometimes in trabeculae of epithelium which may be present in the underlying fibrous connective tissue. The latter is diffusely infiltrated with chronic inflammatory cells – lymphocytes and plasma cells. Many dilated blood vessels adjoin the basal layer of the epithelium. In the mature apical cyst the epithelium assumes an even thickness and may become keratinized, although even so it does not take on the special characteristics of the keratocyst lining. Goblet cells, hyaline bodies (Rushton 1955, Morgan and Johnson 1974), and granular bodies may be found within the lining. Inflammatory cells tend to disappear and fewer capillaries are evident. Clefts left by cholesterol crystals can be seen in the fibrous tissue wall and are surrounded by foreign body giant cells. Occasionally columnar epithelium is observed in the lining membrane of the periodontal cyst.

Secondary infection of a cyst leads to alteration in the epithelial structure, which may take one of the following forms: shrinkage, obliteration or hyperplasia.

Treatment

The most commonly applied procedure in the treatment of apical periodontal cysts is enucleation. This technique is described fully in Chapter 6. The lining of infected cysts may be quite friable and have marked adherence to bone. Several adjoining tooth roots may protrude into the thickness of the lining and through the bony cavity, and preoperative vitality testing of these teeth is essential to exclude those which are sound. Non-vital incriminated teeth are either extracted or, if retention is desirable, are root-filled and, if necessary, an apicectomy performed. An established external sinus track must be excised. In treating large maxillary periodontal cysts, Snawdon (1950, 1957) advised that in all cases there should be provision for permanent drainage either via the floor of the nose or through the outer nasal wall in the meatus, together with closure of the intraoral incision. Snawdon's procedure is discussed in the general chapter on treatment.

Some authorities advise marsupialization when there is a possibility of traumatic penetration of the maxillary sinus and the nose or involvement of the inferior dental nerve (Fig. 8.4). The authors' views on this particular aspect are also given in Chapter 6. To avoid the risk of prejudicing the nerve and vascular supply to adjacent healthy teeth, the roots of which have been denuded of bone by a periodontal cyst, preliminary marsupialization is advocated. Marsupialization is probably the method of choice when treatment is unavoidable in the old and debilitated patient. An important disadvantage of marsupialization is protracted bone regeneration. Another is the risk of occasionally leaving *in situ* neoplastic tissue. This is probably more theoretical than real if an adequate specimen is taken for biopsy and careful follow-up is instituted.

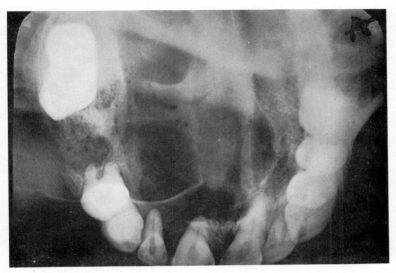

Fig. 8.4 A standard occlusal film of an extensive maxillary cyst. Bony expansion can be seen in the gap between the /4 and /7. The cyst was treated by marsupialization and the opening was made into the wall of the lesion in the area of the gap. Through this window the apices of the majority of the involved upper teeth could be seen projecting into the cyst space. Following operation and the fitting of a suitable bung the cyst cavity gradually became obliterated. After a period of two and a half years only a small depression remained at the site of marsupialization.

Whichever form of treatment is chosen for a periodontal cyst, the patient's affected jaw should be radiographed periodically to confirm that steady bone regeneration is taking place, and follow-ups should be maintained until reversion to a normal bone pattern is complete. This recall arrangement will also ensure that any regrowth – due to the retention of a fragment of cyst membrane – will not be overlooked. For obvious reasons large numbers of films should not be taken at frequent intervals. No harm will ensue, however, from the taking of two or three views, initially at three-monthly intervals and then six-monthly or annually as necessary. This principle will, of course, also apply to review procedures following operation on any type of jaw cyst.

There are two additional aspects concerning treatment which should be noted – aspiration and natural healing. With regard to the former, regular aspiration of the fluid content of a periodontal cyst has been employed abroad as a compromise therapeutic technique (Chipps 1959). The rationale is based on the assumption that the expansile potential of a cyst is arrested temporarily by rupture of its wall, and it is hoped that repeated puncture and drainage will not only curb growth but may even abort the lesion. Apart from the obvious disadvantages of this procedure – that it is time-consuming and does not permit examination of the cyst tissue by a pathologist – it is questionable whether full regression could be achieved since the orifice made in the cyst capsule becomes occluded quite rapidly. After aspiration the cyst fluid is replaced within a short period of time of the puncture healing. It is doubtful if aspiration can be performed sufficiently frequently over a long enough period of time for this to be a practical way of dealing with cysts. What is more, there is the risk of introducing infection at each puncture.

According to Worth (1963), many small periodontal cysts will heal without surgical intervention after the removal of the culpable root or tooth. Most endodontists can cite instances in which periapical lesions of between one and two centimetres diameter have healed after simple root canal treatment and root filling. However, healing does not always follow treatment of the causative tooth.

Reference to natural healing of cysts has also been made. Hayward and Arentz (1963) surmised that necrotizing infections within a cystic cavity might partially or completely destroy the epithelial lining and be followed by bone repair and elimination of the defect. Other theories are considered on page 89.

In a survey of the behaviour of 227 periodontal and residual cysts, Molyneux (1964) found that specific structural changes of an atrophic nature had occurred in the specimens obtained from one group of patients, and he argued that this indicated a quiescent phase and regression in cyst growth. Such considerations, though interesting, are only occasionally relevant to patient treatment, and in general the only realistic curative methods for cysts continue to be enucleation and marsupialization.

Residual cyst

When a periodontal cyst is overlooked after the extraction of the causative permanent tooth or root, it can continue to enlarge and assumes the name of residual cyst.

The alternative processes which can result in the occurrence of a residual cyst are as follows:

1. A small cyst developing upon either a deciduous tooth or a retained root which later exfoliates or is extracted without knowledge of the underlying pathological condition.

2. If the tooth associated with a lateral dentigerous cyst is removed but the existence of the cyst is unrecognized so that it persists and increases in size.

3. Incomplete removal of a periapical cyst or possibly a granuloma.

Typically, the cyst is present in an edentulous area, and the majority of patients are middle-aged or elderly. Incidence is greater in the maxilla than in the mandible.

Resolution of residual cysts with intact linings occasionally occurs but it takes several years.

The mechanism which results in resolution is not clear, but the following suggestions are made:

1. Marsupialization via an empty socket. Radiographic and clinical evidence to support this occurrence is seen from time to time.

2. A repair process including epithelial atrophy (Oehlers 1970).

3. The rupture of the cyst lining during extraction, perhaps with the tearing of part of the lining from the wall of the bony cavity. Organization of the blood clot might establish lymphatic drainage of the cavity and hence resolution of the cyst. It will be recalled that Toller maintains that it is lack of lymphatic access which is a major factor in sustaining an expansile pressure within the cyst.

Treatment

The technique for removal is the same as that employed for an apical cyst, but it is important to preserve the contour of the edentulous ridge.

Lateral radicular (periodontal) cyst

Some cysts developing in relation to the side of the root of a tooth arise as a result of stimulation of epithelial debris of Mallasez by a pulpless tooth. The only difference from the apical radicular cyst is that the communication between the root canal and the periodontal membrane passes out sideways through the root. It may be either a lateral root canal, or an artificial perforation produced during an attempt at root treatment. The condition is to be distinguished from the so-called developmental lateral periodontal cysts which are described in Chapter 8. Treatment follows the principles laid down for the apical radicular cyst.

Lateral periodontal cysts

There is frequently some confusion between lateral radicular cysts, otherwise called lateral (inflammatory) periodontal cysts, and lateral (developmental) periodontal cysts. The former are cysts arising from epithelial debris of Malassez as a result of the presence of a pulpless tooth. They differ in no way from the apical radicular cysts found in relation to pulpless teeth except that they are sited opposite a lateral communication between the root canal and the periodontal membrane (Fig. 8.5). The latter are found lateral to the roots of teeth with vital pulps.

Even when the lateral periodontal cysts are separated from the lateral radicular it may be that the group is not homogeneous but contains several entities.

Lateral periodontal cysts may be found adjacent to the roots of the mandibular third molar. Some are adjacent to the bifurcation of the roots and are either buccal or lingual to the tooth. The lingual ones seem to be the more common and if infected can give rise to an unpleasantly severe spreading infection of the submandibular space. Other examples are found against the distal aspect of the tooth. Seward (1964) affirms that they can be distinguished from the lateral dentigerous cyst because the centre of the cyst cavity lies at a lower level (Fig. 8.6). Further, the lamina dura is destroyed even by a small lateral periodontal cyst while it persists for some considerable time in the case of a lateral dentigerous cyst.

There is uniform agreement that the other site most frequently involved is the canine and premolar region, with the incidence higher in the mandible than the maxilla. Some cysts occur buccal to the tooth concerned and present as a small fluctuant swelling of the masticatory mucosa or at-

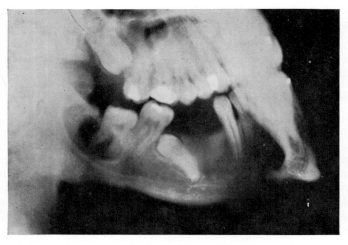

Fig. 8.5 Lateral oblique radiograph of a developmental lateral periodontal cyst in relation to 8/.

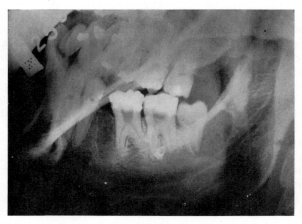

Fig. 8.6 This lateral oblique radiograph reveals a lateral periodontal cyst of developmental type related to the distal root of the lower third molar.

tached gingiva. Such cysts are frequently described as gingival cysts, but Moskow *et al.* (1970) feel that once the thin buccal cortical plate has been penetrated and the cyst involves the periodontal membrane of the adjacent tooth it is impossible to distinguish between gingival and lateral periodontal cysts.

There are a number of possible modes of origin for lateral periodontal cysts. Those which occur opposite to the bifurcation of the roots of the lower third molars could develop in the way demonstrated by Hodson (1957). His specimen shows a cyst developing in continuity with a cord of epithelium arising from the reduced enamel epithelium some distance from the cervical margin of a lower third molar. Such a cord could be considered to be analogous to dental lamina destined to produce a third dentition. The cyst then, by definition, would be a primordial cyst, but it was acutely inflamed and this might account for the fact that it did not exhibit the typical keratocyst lining. Enamel pearls are unusually common on lower third molars (Pedlar 1950) and the proliferation of enamel organ epithelium producing these might be related to such cysts. Colby *et al.* (1961) have suggested a relationship between third molar lateral periodontal cysts and chronic pericoronal inflammation. Such a mechanism would mean an origin from the epithelial debris of Malassez and chronic periodontal inflammation has been suggested by Robinson *et al.* (1951). However, it would not be difficult for such cysts to become infected and drain via the gingival sulcus, so presenting like a periodontal abscess (Cross 1954).

Main (1970) prefers to call lateral periodontal cysts 'collateral primordial cysts' and he believes, like Soskolne and Shear (1967) and Standish and Shafer (1958) that they are a form of keratocyst. There is no doubt that some primordial cysts with typical keratocyst linings do arise in the canine and premolar area of the jaws and, therefore, produce a 'lateral periodontal' type of appearance in radiographs. However, by no means all the cysts which present with this particular radiographic appearance have the keratocyst lining even if they are uninfected.

Another explanation for cysts in the canine premolar region of the jaw is that they are residual radicular cysts from the primary dentition (Figs. 8.7 and 8.8). Stafne (1937 and 1969) favours this explanation. Certainly, retained roots of primary molars which have been separated by resorption from the crown may be found from time to time buried in the interdental bone between the premolars so that the location is right. Radicular cysts on retained and carious primary tooth roots also may be seen in the canine and premolar regions. It would be easy for such cysts to remain as residual cysts if the root were exfoliated, or extracted without the cyst being suspected. Stafne (1969) also makes the point that epithelial rests from the primary dentition may be identified in the same region. He postulates that cysts could develop from these. Whilst this might be a possibility it would seem likely that they would form keratocysts and would be classified as primordial cysts. If the explanation that some of these cysts are residual radicular cysts from the primary dentition is accepted, then the predilection for the canine-- premolar region is readily explained.

The histological appearance of the lining from the cysts is variable. Some are lined by a stratified squamous epithelium and filled with debris outlining cholesterol clefts. Others are lined by a thin, unkeratinized lining of cuboidal cells some two or three cells thick. A thickening of the lining, again of polyhedral and cuboidal cells, may be seen in certain specimens. Yet others have the characteristic keratocyst lining and are probably best classified as primordial cysts, as suggested by Main.

Simple enucleation is indicated, taking care not to damage the roots of adjacent teeth or unduly to disturb their supporting bone. In particular a flap must be reflected from the cervical margins of the adjacent teeth so that the crest of the alveolar bone may be identified and preserved.

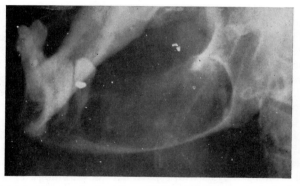

Fig. 8.7 A lateral oblique projection of a residual periodontal cyst in the body of the mandible.

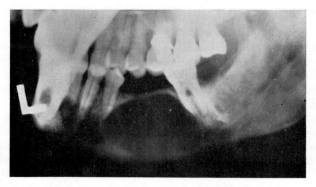

Fig. 8.8 Lateral oblique radiograph of an oval-shaped residual periodontal cyst which has breached the inferior dental canal. Although the lamina dura is partly missing around the roots of the two teeth bordering the lesion, both proved to be vital.

Gingival cysts

Two types of cyst may be classified as gingival cysts. There is the small cyst which protrudes laterally from the gingiva of the adult, and the small lesions known as Bohn's nodules which are seen on the crest of the ridge in the neonate. Small cysts may be found in the gingivae in the adult gingivectomy specimens. Many of these are in the interdental papillae. They are like small keratocysts and it is not known if they ever increase in size to an extent that they are detectable clinically. Some of the ones seen laterally on the gingival mucosa are similar in nature and may be external to the bone or may no more than indent it. Other cysts lateral to the teeth penetrate to the periodontal membrane and are classified with lateral periodontal cysts.

Bohn's nodules are usually small, white nodules similar to the Epstein's pearls seen in the midline of the palate. Some, however, reach 2 mm or so in diameter and take on a pale violet colour because of their contained fluid. They are not uncommon in negro children. They soon disappear and require no treatment. They form small pedunculated swellings on the crest of the ridge and are to be distinguished from cysts of eruption which form an expansion of the gum and occur much later in the child's life. Cysts of eruption are seen mostly in the $1\frac{1}{2}$ to 3-year-old age group over erupting primary molars.

Dentigerous cysts

The term 'dentigerous cyst' was originally used by Paget (1863) for cysts containing teeth and occurring in the jaws. Jourdain (1778) described examples of dentigerous cyst but not under this name, and Heath (1868) distinguished between cysts connected with the roots of fully developed and diseased teeth and cysts connected with imperfectly developed teeth. He would puncture the cyst wall and probe within it in an attempt to detect the presence of a buried tooth.

With the advent of radiography the diagnosis of dentigerous cyst could be made on the radiographic appearances. If a substantial cavity in the jaw surrounded the crown of an unerupted tooth, this was described as a dentigerous cyst. That not all such radiographs represented a simple dentigerous cyst was soon realized. Ameloblastomas and other odontogenic tumours may have a dentigerous relationship to an unerupted tooth. However, in the majority of instances the bone cavity was occupied by a cyst and the diagnostic assumption was justified.

Bennett (1914) recognized that in not every instance, when the cavity of the cyst was opened, was the crown of the tooth to be seen within the cyst cavity. In some cases the tooth was covered by a layer of soft tissue and lay outside the lining. Gillette and Weinmann (1958) described the histological appearance of such cysts, referring to them as extrafollicular cysts, the term used by Seward (1964) in his classification. Toller (1967) refers to these cysts as secondary dentigerous cysts and Browne (1971) as pseudodentigerous cysts. It is now recognized that extrafollicular dentigerous cysts have the keratocyst type of lining. Bennett (1914) suggested an origin for these cysts from the tooth band outside the follicle; an explanation which now proves to be consistent with their histological appearance.

Follicular odontome was another term introduced by Bland-Sutton (1887). He used the term to indicate that the cysts arose from the tooth follicle. This terminology was elaborated and follicular cysts were subdivided into dentigerous cysts and simple follicular cysts, these being cysts not associated with a pulpless tooth and which did not contain the crown of a tooth. Such cysts were subsequently renamed primordial cysts.

Malassez (1885 and 1887) recognized that dentigerous cysts were derived from the epithelial remnants of the enamel organ. Tomes (1873) explained the mechanism of formation of dentigerous cysts as follows:

'When development of the enamel of a tooth is completed, its outer surface becomes perfectly detached and a small quantity of transparent fluid collects in the interval so formed. If the eruption of the tooth is prevented, this fluid gradually increases to distend the surrounding tissues and form a cyst.'

He goes on to compare dentigerous cysts with eruption cysts and concludes that they are of the same nature.

The plane at which the tissues separate from the crown of the tooth is still uncertain. Lartschneider's contention that the fluid separates the follicle from the bare surface of the enamel (Lartschneider 1929), other than in a macroscopic sense, has been challenged by Toller (1967). He reports sectioning some 15 teeth from dentigerous cysts using a double embedding technique and reports that Nasmyth's membrane still covered the crowns of 13 out of the 15.

McHugh (1961) describes the maturation of the reduced enamel epithelium and eruption of the tooth. After the deposition of the primary enamel cuticle the ameloblasts are seen as columnar cells with more centrally placed nuclei. Over them is a layer of squamous type cells of varying thickness with capillaries in the indentations. The ameloblasts become reduced to a cuboidal shape and their nuclei become pyknotic. As the tooth approaches the surface the outer layer proliferates and the ameloblasts become flattened and degenerate. At the same time the overlying mucosal epithelium proliferates and ceases to keratinize, and a dimple forms at the future site of penetration. The two proliferating masses approach one another and fuse to form the gingival cuff. Even before penetration of the surface by the tip of the cusp the epithelium splits between the gingival cuff epithelium and the degenerating ameloblast layer. This split extends around the crown to form the gingival crevice and the degenerate ameloblasts form the secondary examel cuticle. The process of proliferation of the outer layer of the reduced enamel epithelium and fusion with proliferating gingival cuff cells extends down the tooth towards the cervical margin, accompanied by degeneration of the ameloblasts and extension of the gingival crevice split. Harris (1974) suggests that the experimental follicular cysts of Bartlett *et al.* (1973) arise by the programmed formation of the crevicular split.

A further possibility is that the connective tissue of the follicle separates from the reduced enamel epithelium, perhaps with the adhesion of some epithelium cells in certain places. Either by proliferation of these foci of epithelium, or by proliferation of reduced enamel epithelium cells at the periphery of the separation, the surface would become covered with epithelium. Certainly the presence of simple epithelial discontinuities in the lining of both radicular and dentigerous cysts (Toller 1966) shows that an intact epithelial layer is not essential for the growth and persistence of a cyst. Consideration of solitary bone cysts which have no lining epithelium suggest further that an epithelial layer is not essential for the initiation of a cyst.

Clinical observation demonstrates that the tooth follicle separates readily from the crown of an unerupted tooth. At the time of eruption of the primary dentition the overlying gum becomes hyperaemic and swollen. Should there be a need to incise the mucosa over the tooth at this stage a small quantity of fluid may be released as described by Tomes (1873), and a plane of cleavage is uncovered between the overlying soft tissues and the crown. If it is accepted that the cyst of eruption, seen so commonly over erupting primary molars, is a comparable process to the formation of a dentigerous cyst, then again it is found that the soft tissues are separated from the macroscopically bare surface of the tooth crown by a collection of fluid. Section of the overlying soft tissue may, or may not, demonstrate a thin layer of epithelium on the cavity aspect. In support of Harris's contention it can be argued that as cysts of eruption are so common over the primary molars, and generally no impediment to the eruption of the tooth, they are merely a florid expression of the normal processes of tooth eruption.

In 1924, Mummery commented upon the pigmentation of the surface and subsurface enamel in the incisal two-thirds of a canine from a dentigerous cyst. It is generally agreed that development of the crowns of teeth involved in dentigerous cysts is complete, and usually there is no gross defect of their surface enamel. However, Crabb (1963) demonstrated more subtle changes in four teeth from dentigerous cysts. He noted zones of subsurface layer demineralization which coincided in order and characteristics with those produced by the early lesions of caries. He remarked that the zones did not correspond with the sequence of mineralization of the enamel, suggesting that they resulted from attack by some component of cyst fluid. Harris (1974) speculated about this process in relationship to enzymes produced by the follicle during the eruption of teeth and the presence of prostaglandins.

From time to time it has been proposed that dentigerous cysts arise as a result of secondary involvement of unerupted teeth by cysts arising adjacent to them. Colyer and Sprawson (1942) were proponents of the concept that dentigerous cysts involving canines and premolars were due to radicular cysts on carious deciduous predecessors. Some dentigerous cysts on third molars, they thought, arose in a similar fashion from carious first molars; the rest being enlarged cysts of eruption. In practice, a few dentigerous cysts are seen around the crowns of premolars and in relationship to grossly carious primary molars above them. The crown of the premolar is not covered by soft tissue and has a true (primary) dentigerous relationship to the premolar. The part played by the carious deciduous tooth therefore remains obscure and a number of possible relationships can be enumerated. The inflammatory reaction local to a maturing premolar tooth might accelerate the programmed changes in the enamel epithelium and increase the amount of fluid produced in the gingival crevice split. Resorption of the infected primary tooth might be delayed and out of phase with maturation of the underlying tooth germ. Perhaps a radicular cyst develops on the apices of the primary tooth and the epithelium is treated like gingival epithelium with fusion of its basal layers to the reduced enamel epithelium of the successional tooth and 'eruption' of the tooth into the cyst cavity.These entities apart, most dentigerous cysts have no relationship to a pulpless tooth and the general contention of involvement by a radicular cyst is not applicable. Indeed, in general, secondary involvement of an unerupted tooth by a cyst is distinguishable radiographically for an appreciable time (Seward 1956). The bony margin of both the follicular space and the gubernacular canal of the unerupted tooth remain visible radiographically. In contrast, the follicular space outline of the extrafollicular dentigerous cyst is destroyed early, indicating that the epithelium involved lies very close to the outside of the fibrous layer of the follicle, since this remains intact histologically.

It is now possible to rationalize the uses of the various terms. 'Dentigerous cyst', therefore, is a clinical term for cysts which (radiographically) cause an enlargement of the follicular space about the whole, or part of the crown of the tooth. On the result of observations at operation, or at the histological examination of the specimen, extrafollicular dentigerous cysts can be distinguished from primary dentigerous cysts. Primary dentigerous cysts are lined by cells derived from the reduced enamel epithelium and are the major concern of this chapter. Cysts of eruption also are lined by cells derived from the reduced enamel epithelium, but generally involve teeth with no deciduous predecessor and produce no significant changes in the alveolar bone. They are normally transient and rupture spontaneously.

Extrafollicular dentigerous cysts, like primordial cysts, are keratocysts. The former are clinical terms describing what is seen in the patient and in the radiographs. 'Keratocyst' is a term related to the histopathological appearance of the lining. It is understood to imply development of the cyst from part of the dental lamina. It is suggested, therefore, that extrafollicular dentigerous cysts develop from the 'glands of Serres'. These are the remnants of the dental lamina immediately above the enamel organ.

A primary dentigerous cyst is formed in relationship to a normal permanent tooth, but rarely it may be associated with a supernumerary tooth, or a complex or composite odontome. Dentigerous cysts related to double impactions of molar teeth are usually of the extrafollicular type. Several positional variations of cyst to tooth have been described and are of interest, although not of great clinical significance. Most commonly the cyst is central or pericoronal, enveloping the crown symmetrically and producing pressure upon its occlusal surface so that the tooth may be forced apically in a direction opposite to its normal eruptive movement. The cyst may have a tangential connection to the tooth, i.e. developing on the medial or lateral aspect with an attachment at the amelocemental junction, but with only one side of the crown in direct apposition to the cyst cavity. Genesis of the lateral type is ascribed to the splitting of the reduced enamel epithelium along one side of the crown of the tooth. In fact a narrow slit-like cavity frequently extends around the rest of the crown, and more subtle factors are probably involved. Typically a lateral

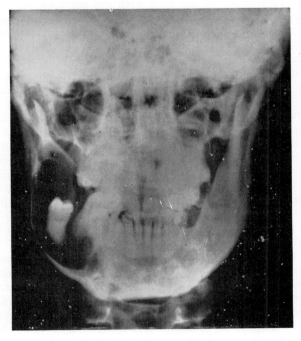

Fig. 8.9 Postero-anterior radiograph of a large dentigerous cyst associated with a third molar which has involved the ramus and angle and extended forwards into the body of the mandible.

dentigerous cyst is found in association with a lower third molar (Fig. 8.9), and although it may not obstruct the eruptive progress of that tooth, especially if related distally, nevertheless, the third molar may be deviated from its normal path in a direction away from the involved side. Distally placed dentigerous cysts may undergo spontaneous resolution.

Dentigerous cysts occur in the mandible more frequently than in the maxilla. Teeth which erupt late are those most often concerned in dentigerous cyst formation, and in numerical order of occurrence these are the mandibular third molar, the maxillary canine and the mandibular second premolar. Other teeth in the normal dentition are occasionally involved as well as supernumeraries, and certain developmental anomalies of the teeth and hamartomas of the dental tissues.

In most cases only one dentigerous cyst is found, but examples are encountered of multiple dentigerous cysts of lower first molars. The phenomena of bilateral third molar cysts may have a familial tendency separate from instances of the multiple cyst–basal cell naevus syndrome. Indeed the dentigerous cysts in the latter instance are usually of the extrafollicular variety.

The incidence appears to be equal in the two sexes and the commonest age periods for diagnosis are childhood and adolescence. The rate of growth of the cystic condition in the bone of a child is rapid, and cysts of 4 to 5 cm in diameter will be found to have developed in three to four years according to the radiographic calculations of Seward (1964). In adults dentigerous cyst enlargement is much slower.

From the effect of pressure, it is possible for the tooth of origin at the periphery of the cystic lesion to migrate a considerable distance. In the body of the mandible it may come to occupy a position near to the inferior border (Fig. 8.10), and in the ramus to reach the mandibular notch. In the upper jaw, expansion may move the tooth upwards as high as the floor of the orbit, or deflect it in an anterior direction so that it lies beneath the floor of the nose. Maxillary third molars travel up the posterior wall and canines up the anterior wall of the maxillary sinus. Adjacent developing teeth encroached upon by the growing cyst may also be displaced, and in the lower jaw forced to remain at the inferior margin of the lesion.

Clinical findings

Often the cyst is extensive before discovery, so that it is a progressive facial asymmetry that induces the patient to seek advice. A tooth will be missing from the permanent series unless an unsuspected supernumerary or complex odontome is responsible. Sometimes other adjacent involved teeth also fail to erupt or the roots of adjoining teeth may be tilted (Fig. 8.11). Pain may be a symptom if infection supervenes. A denture wearer's first intimation that something is wrong may be a sudden or gradual alteration in the fit of the denture. The other features are similar to those found in patients with radicular cysts.

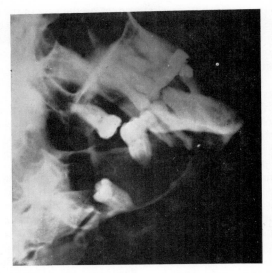

Fig. 8.10 Lateral oblique film of a large dentigerous cyst in the ramus and body of the mandible which has displaced the molar into an aberrant position.

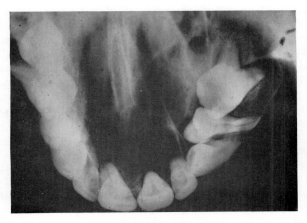

Fig. 8.11 An occlusal view showing a large maxillary cyst. The /6 is unerupted and the roots of /45 are tilted.

Radiological examination

If the cyst remains clinically dormant, its presence will be recognized only as an accidental finding on routine radiography. Essentially a unilocular bone cavity is seen associated with the crown of an unerupted tooth. Occasionally ostensible multilocularity is seen, but the appearance is not due to true septa, but merely to ridges on the wall of the cavity. The margin of the bony cavity is well defined, but not necessarily demarcated by a white line. Where the jaw is expanded the cyst is covered by a layer of subperiosteal new bone. Resorption of the roots of adjacent teeth occurs more often than was believed in the past.

Cyst contents
Yellowish fluid exudes from the cyst sac on penetration of the wall. Cholesterol crystals may be identified microscopically, and if the cyst is acutely infected the fluid may be purulent.

Histological appearance
The cyst lining is usually attached to the tooth at the amelocemental junction and the sac lined by a thin, regular, stratified squamous epithelium. It seems probable that some primary dentigerous cysts are lined by a parakeratinized or keratinized lining, without having the other characteristics of keratocysts. Up to three per cent may be lined with mucous cells. Hyaline bodies may be seen within the epithelium and clefts from cholesterol crystals in the connective tissue capsule. These may be outlined by foreign body giant cells. Simple epithelial discontinuities and discontinuities due to the discharge of cholesterol into the lumen may be seen.

Sometimes macroscopic examination of the inner surface of the removed cyst reveals small mural thickenings which, on microscopic examination, contain proliferating odontogenic epithelium. These strands may exhibit follicular enlargements and can resemble ameloblastomas. Conversely, some ameloblastomas have a dentigerous relationship to an unerupted tooth. If the ameloblastoma forms a fairly solid tumour mass about the crown of the tooth the true diagnosis is unlikely to be missed. If it forms a large unilocular cyst there is a risk that the true character of the lining tissue will not be appreciated.

Treatment
Marsupialization as a method of treatment in children is satisfactory, provided a suitably wide opening can be made into the cyst and provided an adequate specimen of lining is sent for histological examination. The rapid formation of new bone will cause the cavity to shrink in size and both the tooth of origin and any other teeth which were prevented from eruption by the cyst will move upwards through the jaw (Fig. 8.12).

Orthodontic treatment may be necessary to prevent loss of space in the arch and to correct the alignment of the teeth. Satisfactory eruption of the tooth and obliteration of the cavity is far less likely to follow marsupialization during adult life. Some shrinkage of the cyst, however, may reduce the risk of jaw fracture during removal of the teeth where initially the cavity was very large.

Alternatively the cyst can be enucleated. If this is done the tooth of

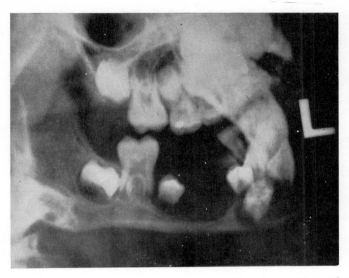

Fig. 8.12 Radiographic appearance of a dentigerous cyst in a young patient. After marsupialization of the cyst the teeth involved erupted normally.

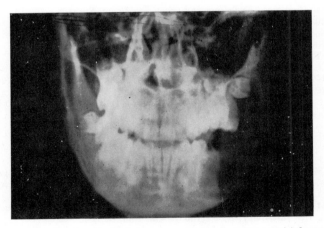

Fig. 8.13 Radiograph of a dentigerous cyst occupying the ramus and left angle of the mandible. The /78 have been displaced into the coronoid process.

origin is usually removed with the lining in the adult. In children an attempt may be made to conserve the tooth, but it is necessary to separate the lining from the neck of tooth with a scalpel. Even so, should little of the root have formed there is a considerable risk that the tooth will be dislodged (Figs. 8.13 and 8.14).

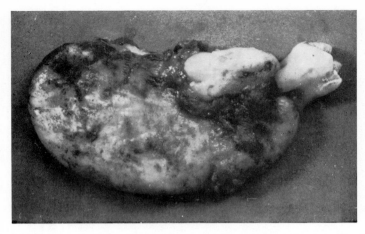

Fig. 8.14 Cyst sac and associated teeth removed from the area shown in Fig. 8.13.

REFERENCES

Alberran, (1888) *Revie de Chir.*
Bartlett, P. F., Radden B. G. & Redde, P. C. (1973) *J. Oral Path.,* **2,** 58.
Bennett, N. C. (1914) *The Science and Practice of Dental Surgery.* Oxford Univ. Press.
Bland-Sutton, J. (1917) *Tumours Innocent and Malignant,* 6th ed. London: Cassell.
Bland-Sutton, J. (1889) *Trans. Odont. Soc.,* **XV,** 185.
Bland-Sutton, J. (1887) *Trans. Odont. Soc.,* **XX,** 34.
Browne, R. M. (1971) *Brit. dent. J.,* **131,** 249.
Chipps, J. E. (1959) *Dent. Clin. N. Am.,* Nov., 755.
Colby, R. A., Kerr, D. A. & Robinson, H. B. G. (1961) *Colour Atlas of Oral Pathology,* 2nd ed. London: Pitman.
Colyer, J. F. & Sprawson, E. (1942) *Dental Surgery & Pathology,* 8th ed. London: Longman.
Cowan, A. (1953) *Dent. Practic.,* **3,** 130.
Crabb, H. S. M. (1963) *Brit. dent. J.,* **114,** 499.
Cross, W. G. (1954) *J. Periodont.,* **25,** 287.
Gillette, P. & Weinmann, J. P. (1958) *Oral Surg.,* **11,** 638.
Harris, M. (1974) Prostaglandin reduction and bone resorption by dental cysts. Hunterian lecture at the Royal College of Surgeons of England, 15 March.
Harris, M. & Goldhaber, (1973) *Br. J. Oral Surg.,* **10,** 334.
Harris, M., Jenkins, M. B., Bennett, A. & Wills, M. R. (1973) *Nature,* **245,** 213.
Hayward, J. R. & Arentz, R. E. (1963) *Dent. Clin. N. Am.,* March, 127.
Heath, C. (1868) *Injuries and Disease of the Jaws.* London: Churchill.
Hodson, J. J., (1956) *Proc. Roy. Soc. Med.,* **49,** 637.
Ingram, F. (1965) *Radiology of the Teeth and Jaws,* 2nd ed. London: Arnold.
Jourdain, A. (1778) *Traite des Maladies de la Bouche,* vol. 1, p. 119. Paris: Vallegre.
Lartschneider, J. (1929) *Dental Cosmos,* **71,** 788.
Ledingham, J. C. (1933) *J. Path. Bact.,* **34,** 123.
Livingston, A. (1927) *Dent. Rec.,* **47,** 531.
McHugh, W. D. (1961) *Dent. Practit.,* **11,** 314.
Main, D. M. G. (1970) *Brit. J. oral Surg.,* **8,** 114.
Malassez, L. C. (1887) *Comptes Rendus de la Societe de Biologie Serie VIII.*

Malassez, L. C. (1885) *Archiv de Physiologie Serie III*, **V**, 129.
Molyneux, G. S. (1964) *Oral Surg.*, **10**, 75.
Morgan, P. R. & Johnson, N. W. (1974) *J. Oral Path.*, **3**, 127.
Moskow, B. S., Siegel, K., Zegarelli, E. V., Kutscher, A. H. & Rothenberg, F. (1970). *J. Periodontol.*, **41**, 249.
Mummery, J. H. (1924) *Brit. dent. J.*, **45**, 620.
Oehlers, F. A. C. (1970) *Brit. J. oral Surg.*, **8**, 103.
Paget, J. (1863) *Lectures in Surgical Pathology*, 2nd ed. London: Longman.
Pedler, (195?)
Powell-White, C. (1910) *J. Path. Bact.*, **14**, 45.
Robinson, H. B. G., Koch, W. E. and Kolas, S. (1956) *Dent. Radiog. Photog.*, **29**, 61.
Rushton, M. A. (1955), *Proc. Roy. Soc. Med.*, 407.
Rushton, M. A. & Cooke, B. E. D. (1959) *Oral Histopathology*. Edinburgh: Livingstone.
Sealey, V. T. (1948), *Aust. J. Dent.*, **52**, 244.
Seltzer, S., Soltanoff, W. and Bender, I. B., (1969), *Oral Surg.*, **27**, 111.
Seward, G. R. (1964) *Brit. dent. J.*, **115**, 175.
Seward, G. R. (1963) *Brit. dent. J.*, **115**, 229.
Seward, G. R. (1956) *Dent. Practit.*, **6**, 212.
Seward, M. H. (1973) *J. oral Surg.*, **31**, 31.
Shear, M. (1963) *Dent. Practit.*, **13**, 238.
Snawdon, J. W. E (1957) *Int. dent. J.*, **7**, 493.
Snawdon, J. W. E. (1950) *Dent. Practit*, **1**, 105.
Sonesson, A. (1950) *Acta Radiol.* Suppl. 81.
Soskolne, W. A. & Shear, M. (1967) *Brit. dent. J.*, **123**, 321.
Stafne, E. C. (1942) *J. Am. Dent. Ass.*, **29**, 1969.
Stafne, E. C. (1969) *Oral Roentgenographic Diagnosis*, 3rd ed. Philadelphia: Saunders.
Standish, S. M. & Shafer, W. G. (1958) *J. Periodontol.*, **29**, 27.
Stokke, T. (1956) *Acta Odont. Scand.*, **14**, 65.
Ten-Cate, A. R. (1963) *Arch. Oral Biol.*, **8**, 755.
Ten-Cate, A. R. (1972) *Oral Surg.*, **34**, 956.
Thoma, K. H. (1964) *Oral Surg.*, **18**, 368.
Toller, P. A. (1970) *Brit. dent. J.*, **128**, 317.
Toller, P. A. (1967) *Ann. Roy. Col. Surg. of Eng.*, **40**, 306.
Toller, P. A. (1966) *Brit. dent. J.*, **120**, 74.
Toller, P. A. (1948) *Proc. R. Soc. Med.*, **41**, 681.
Tomes, C. (1873) *Dental Surgery*
Tratman, E. K. (1939), *Brit. Dent. J.*, **66**, 515.
Valderhaug, J. (1972), *Int. J. Oral Surg.*, **1**, 137.
Walter, J. B. & Israel, M. S. (1974), *General Pathology*, 4th ed. Edinburgh: Churchill Livingstone.
Worth, H. M. (1963) *Principles and Practice of Oral Radiographic Interpretation*. Chicago: Year Book.

9. Non-Odontogenic Cysts

Fissural cysts

The cysts which are classified as fissural or non-odontogenic in origin are alleged to arise from epithelial inclusions at the line of closure of embryonic processes of from vestigial epithelial remains. The individual designation of each cyst is related to its anatomical location.

In recent years a clearer understanding of embryological development has cast doubt upon the origin of a number of cysts previously considered to be fissural or non-odontogenic. It has been necessary therefore to re-examine the evidence for the existence of these cysts, and where necessary, to explain their occurrence in other ways. Chapter 2 sets out in detail the development of the face in relationship to the origin of cysts of the jaws.

Median mandibular cysts

There is no longer a reasonable explanation for the occurrence of cysts at the midline of the mandible on developmental grounds. Median sublingual dermoid cysts are well recognized and may be found immediately lingual to the mandible. Their origin in relation to the development of the tongue may be understood. Epithelium-lined pits may be found in the lower lip as bilateral and paramedian structures, but not as a single median structure. Median mandibular clefts involve a gross separation of the two sides of the mandible and frequently the floor of mouth and the tongue as well. There is no suggestion that these arise as a simple failure of epithelium-covered processes to unite. The origin of median mandibular cysts must be sought elsewhere.

Some are likely to be identified as solitary bone cysts or keratocysts once histological material is available (Fig. 9.1). More careful examination of the two central incisors may show that one is pulpless. However a residuum of cases are not readily explicable in this fashion. Olech (1957), Meyer (1957), Lucchesi and Topazian (1961) and Albers (1973) have reported cases and examined possible explanations for their origin.

Typically these cysts are found in the midline of the mandible and labial to the roots of the standing teeth, which are symmetrically disposed around the periphery. All the adult lower incisors are vital and the cyst is lined with stratified squamous epithelium. They are rarely larger than 1.5 to 2 cm in diameter. A possible explanation for these cysts is that they are residual radicular cysts from a pulpless tooth of the primary dentition.

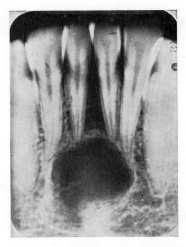

Fig. 9.1 Intraoral radiograph of a bone cavity situated in the lower anterior region which at operation was found to be a solitary bone cyst. The report following pathological examination of a specimen of the enclosing bone supported this diagnosis. All the lower incisors were vital.

Median fissural cysts of the maxilla

There would seem to be every reason to expect median developmental cysts of the palate to exist, because of the manner in which the two palatine processes of the maxilla unite. In fact, no clearly and unequivocally substantiated cases have been described to our knowledge. Median alveolar cysts, anterior to the incisive canals, are also unknown to the authors, and the development of the primary palate as a median structure would not lead us to expect them to exist.

Median clefts of the premaxillary region exist, but these cases are due to failures of development of frontonasal mesenchyme and are related to cyclopia. Failure of epithelium-covered processes to unite is not involved. Indeed in mild cases only a submucous and subcutaneous deficiency exists. Indeed, even if the premaxilla and external nose are absent, there may still be a complete upper lip and upper dental arch, although the incisors will not be present. Other so-called median alveolar clefts are merely due to wide median suture lines between the maxillary bones which are filled with a thick, hyperplastic frenum.

Globulomaxillary cyst

Characteristically the globulomaxillary cyst occupies the bony septum between the maxillary permanent lateral incisor and canine roots (Fig. 9.2). As was explained in Chapter 2, the possibility exists that these could develop from the nasal fin. In practice we feel this is unlikely, or at most,

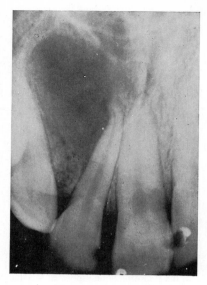

Fig. 9.2 A periapical radiograph of a globulomaxillary cyst showing divergence of the roots of 32/ and approximation of their crowns.

an extremely uncommon event for reasons discussed earlier. Indeed, if illustrations of radiographs of so-called globulomaxillary cysts in most papers and textbooks are examined critically, it is usual to be able to detect a likely cause of death of the pulp of the lateral incisor. A cingulum invagination is frequently to be seen, and as this is not as obvious as a carious cavity or unlined restoration, the loss of vitality of the tooth may well have been overlooked.

If such cases are eliminated, and Seward (1956) has explained how radicular cysts on lateral incisors may involve the septal bone between lateral incisor and canine, then a residue of cases remains in which both teeth have normal vital pulps. Some of these may be keratocysts or developmental periodontal cysts, and in such a case the type of lining characteristic of these entities will be found. Others may be residual radicular cysts from the primary dentition.

Nasopalatine cyst (Figs. 9.3–9.5)

The generic term 'nasopalatine cyst' refers both to the cyst of the incisive canal and the cyst of the palatine papilla. Diversity between the two is based on the premise that the former is intraosseous in origin, but the latter is located solely within the soft tissues in the region of the papilla. However, some authorities do not accept this distinction.

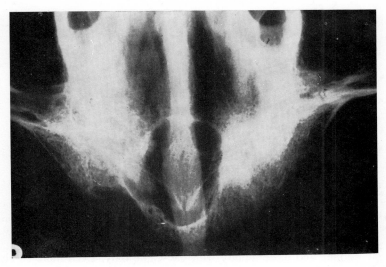

Fig. 9.3 A standard occlusal radiograph of a nasopalatine cyst which is asymmetrically disposed about the midline.

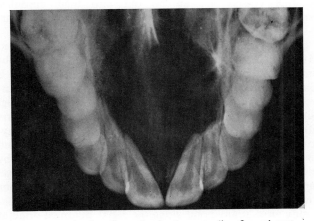

Fig. 9.4 A standard occlusal radiograph of a large median fissural cyst.

Incisive canal cyst

Vestigial cords of epithelium are to be found in the soft tissue contents of the incisive canals and fossa. Epithelium-lined cysts are to be found which occupy deep concavities replacing the normal smaller and shallower incisive fossa. The bony cavity is usually in continuity with both incisive canals but sometimes it is smaller, displaced just to one side

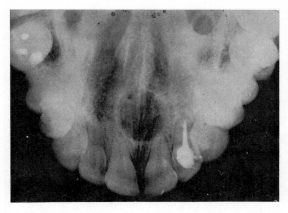

Fig. 9.5 Occlusal radiograph of a typical nasopalatine cyst showing a rounded and well-delineated outline.

of the midline and in continuity with one canal only. Even more rarely there are two cystic compartments, each in continuity with a canal. It is characteristic of these cysts that the long sphenopalatine nerves and sphenopalatine vessels are spread out into their capsules. Most authorities are happy to accept incisive canal cysts as developmental in origin.

In a chapter devoted to non-odontogenic, epithelium-lined cysts, Stafne (1958) claimed that those in the incisive canal were probably the most common, and Seward (1964) subscribes to this opinion. Six hundred cadavers were examined by Meyer (1931) who identified an incisive canal cyst in one out of every 66 specimens studied. An investigation of the incisive fossae in 2394 skulls at the Department of Anthropology, University of Cambridge, was made by one of the authors (Kay) and in only two specimens was there evidence of a cystic enlargement at that site. This finding implies that those cystic lesions detectable by actual enlargement of the incisive fossa are less numerous than suggested by Meyer, and such a contention is supported by the results of a comparable survey by Roper-Hall (1938).

Cysts may arise at any point along the canal, but most originate in the lower portion. Increase in size is slow and they may remain static for many years. It has been suggested that intermittent drainage of fluid content may be responsible for this. Enlargement tends to be limited to a maximum diameter of 2 cm, and this observation is supported by measurements recorded in a series reviewed by Abrahams *et al.* (1963) in which the majority were between 0.6 and 1.5 cm in diameter. It is also substantiated by Kay's findings. Occasionally, however, cysts of this type may attain larger proportions, and the authors have encountered an incisive canal cyst which extended as far posteriorly as the upper first molar and was 4 cm in width.

Aetiology

Many aetiological factors have been advanced to explain the epithelial proliferation which is alleged to lead to cystic development. Trauma to the area of the palatine papilla from mastication or an ill-fitting denture has been suggested. Some believe that extension of bacterial infection through a canal patent either into the nose or into the mouth may encourage growth of a cyst, but in fact such patent vestigial canals are an uncommon finding in this region. Blocked ducts of mucous glands or the accumulation of secretions from a mucus-secreting lining are also proposed as explanations, but do not accord with histological findings. Indeed there is no credible evidence to justify the validity of any of these suggestions.

Clinical findings

Small, blue, submucous swellings may be seen posterior to the palatine papilla in young children of about 3 to 4 years of age. These small, symptomless cysts do not produce radiographically detectable changes and, therefore, could be viewed as incisive papilla cysts. On the other hand, they may represent the incisive canal cyst in this age group. The youngest child with an incisive canal cyst producing the typical radiographic appearance that has been seen by the authors was aged 13. Intrabony incisive canal cysts prior to this age are particularly uncommon, because the upper incisor region of many children is radiographed for orthodontic reasons and such cysts are not encountered as chance findings.

The majority remain asymptomatic, but even when insidious symptoms do arise, they do not follow a consistent pattern and may produce such little disturbance that the condition is tolerated for a long period before treatment is solicited. Indeed, it is not uncommon to find the imprint of a palatal swelling caused by such a cyst on the fitting surface of a full upper denture, showing that it antedated the taking of the impression from which the denture was made.

The most frequent complaint is of a lump in the midline of the palate anteriorly, and on palpation this may be springy in consistency, but more usually it is fluctuant. Palatal expansion is not inevitable, however, and occasionally penetration of the labial plate may take place. This leads to a swelling beneath the upper labial frenum, or to one side of it, close to the root of a central incisor. Secondary infection is responsible for a rapid increase in the swelling and if this occurs on the palatal aspect, it leads to displacement of any denture which covers it. Often infection is accompanied by pain, which is either well localized or neuralgic in character, radiating to the side of the nose or the eyes. Pain is not always related to suppuration, and occasionally a burning sensation is experienced which may be due to pressure transmitted by the cyst to the long sphenopalatine nerves. Occasionally a discharge can be observed, emanating from a sinus opening at or near the papilla, and a track leading to the cyst can be demonstrated by probing. Should an infected cyst rupture through a labial swelling a sinus in the sulcus will result. A salty taste, 'numbness' in the anterior palate and sensations of pressure or fullness with tenderness on palpation in that region are often quoted prominent features of the condition. The adjacent incisors should be normal in colour and not sensitive to percussion, but the percussion note may be dull and the crowns may be tilted slightly towards one another. A periapical abscess or radicular cyst should be excluded by vitality testing of both central incisors. Indeed, a mistaken diagnosis of apical abscess or cyst because of failure to demonstrate the vitality of the adjacent teeth is one of the classical pitfalls of dentistry.

It would be expected that a cyst originating high in the canal would eventually produce nasal symptoms, and in a patient with nasal occlusion seen by Hyde (1942) loss of smell was the predominant complaint.

Radiological examination

In many cases there are no accompanying symptoms, and a fortuitous radiological examination may provide the only indication of cystic development. The radiolucency of the cyst which replaces the normal image of the incisive fossa is frequently circumscribed in outline and symmetrically positioned with regard to the midline. Occasionally the cystic expansion is unilateral in character. Some cysts appear to be heart-shaped and even give the impression of being a form of paired cyst, but the cavity is unilocular and the apparent ridge or septum is due to a superimposition of the radio-opaque images of the buttress of the anterior nasal spine and the septal crest of the pre-maxilla.

The distinction between a small cyst and a normal incisive fossa radiologically is not always easy. A large and deep fossa is normally continuous with wide, funnel-shaped canals, but a cyst may be related either to wide or to narrow canals. The normal fossa is sharply delineated at its lateral margins, but rarely so on its superior (radiographically in periapical films) or palatal margin. The lower or incisal margin also usually lacks sharpness radiographically. Once a cyst develops the fossa becomes a distinct, almost hemispherical, concavity, the palatal aspect of the lining being covered by palatal mucoperiosteum. All aspects of the cavity will now lie tangential to the radiographic beam and produce a well-defined margin. As the cyst increases in size at the expense of the alveolar process, so a more characteristically 'cystic' lesion is revealed in the radiograph. The apices of the central incisors are at first superimposed in oblique periapical views, but the lamina dura image is undisturbed. The periodontal membrane shadow may appear widened due to image 'burn out', but this is an artifact. As the cyst encroaches upon the tooth roots, they are displaced and the outline of the cyst indented at those points. However, again the lamina dura persists for some time and will be visible unless a sizeable example has been encountered. A standard occlusal film is particularly informative on position, and generally will reassure the operator by disclosing that the cyst lies behind the roots of the central incisors.

By contrast, a radicular cyst associated with a central incisor develops to one side of the median plane and the lamina dura around its apex is deficient from the outset. What is more, a vitality test will demonstrate that the tooth is pulpless.

In case of genuine doubt about the differential diagnosis between a deep incisive fossa and a cyst, aspiration is a simple test which will settle the matter. The area is a sensitive one, however, and careful anaesthetization of the tissue is necessary. Alternatively, when faced with the dilemma after routine radiography of deciding whether a cyst is present or the fossa merely a large anatomical variant, it may be prudent to defer surgical exploration and radiograph the suspicious area at regular intervals to determine whether its size remains unaltered or not.

Another problem of differential diagnosis concerns the coincident occurrence of a cyst and a supernumerary. It is not always easy preoperatively to distinguish between an incisive canal cyst and a dentigerous cyst on a mesiodens under these circumstances.

An important point to remember is that radiographic angulation could cause so much distal displacement of the image of a nasopalatine cyst that the radiolucency might be projected over a lateral incisor root. Finally, it is inadvisable to rely on a single view, e.g. a periapical film, alone. Both occlusal and periapical radiographs are necessary for clarification when distortion is suspected, and they are complementary to each other in separating the canal cyst from the other pathological entities. In the case of the edentulous maxilla a tangential view can be most helpful.

Comment – A precise maximum limit cannot be placed upon the size of a normal incisive fossa (anterior palatine foramen) beyond which an increase in dimension would be positive evidence of a pathological process. Even if this were so, it would still be feasible for a cystic condition in early development to be present in the lower part of the incisive canal and escape radiological detection until its expanded diameter exceeded the accepted norm for the X-ray shadow of the fossa. However, it is expedient for diagnostic purposes to define an arbitrary restriction in width for the normal fossa, so that a dimensional increase over that set figure would raise suspicion of abnormality, whilst lack of alteration in size would not necessarily exclude a cystic formation.

In 1938, Roper-Hall scrutinized 2162 skulls and from the results of this survey he concluded that the average transverse diameter of the fossa (width) was 3 mm. The most frequent large-sized fossa was 5 mm wide, 7 mm anteroposteriorly and 5 mm high, but seven normal fossae with measurements greater than this were recorded. The author states that a shadow less than 6 mm in width could be considered within normal limits.

From one of the authors (Kay) own investigation of 2394 fossae, which represented a cross-section of differing nationalities and age periods ranging from ancient to modern times, the most frequent widths were 4.5 and 5 mm, and only two apparently normal cavities exceeded a 6 mm transverse diameter. Using Roper-Hall's criteria, the mean anteroposterior length was 4 mm and the vertical height or depth measured from the level of the posterior palatal edge was on average 3 mm in extent. In two specimens the cavities, which were probably cystic, reached widths of 8 and 9 mm, and the other dimensions were increased beyond the assumed limits for a natural fossa, being respectively 14 and 17 mm anteroposteriorly and 8 and 8.5 mm in height. In six specimens an actual incisive fossa did not exist, but there were minute apertures at the recognized site representing the foramina of the incisive canals.

The findings were in accord with the view of Roper-Hall that age and race have no apparent effect upon the size and position of the fossa. They also provided endorsement of his statement that any radiograph of the fossa which shows a shadow less than 6 mm wide may be considered within normal limits in the absence of specific symptoms. Although it would seem unsatisfactory to rely upon a radiological diameter when a decision on an arbitrary maximum width was reached after dried skull measurements, nevertheless a test comparison of respective diameters reveals that the distortion of fossa size on standard periapical and occlusal films is minimal. It would not seem essential for practical purposes to attempt to allow for a possible slight disparity between the two measurements by computing a magnification or reduction factor.

The contour of normal fossae in the series was circular, elliptical or heart-shaped and dimensionally the antero-posterior length was usually greater than the width. The shape of an incisive canal cyst will be altered only slightly by variation in X-ray projection, whereas the incisive fossa will tend to change in form. Variations in the degree of radiolucency of the fossa are also dependent upon angulation of the direct rays, and the closer the path of the rays is to a parallel with the axial inclination of the canal the darker will be the shadow.

Pathological examination

To recapitulate, most nasopalatine cysts occupy the lower end of the canal but positional variability occurs, and cysts have been reported which originated in the vicinity of the nasal orifice. Although there is not an absolute correlation between cyst site and the type of epithelium found, almost consistently squamous epithelium is seen in cyst linings taken from the inferior portion of the canal, and respiratory epithelial tissue or modifications of it appear above that level. Unexpected diversions from this descending pattern in epithelial type may be due to metaplastic transformation. The transition at different levels may provide examples of cuboidal as well as ciliated and pseudostratified ciliated columnar epithelium. The connective tissue capsule may contain mucous gland tissue. Cartilage too may be identified in the wall of the cyst, but it is surmised that sometimes juxtaposed cartilaginous tissue may be excised inadvertently from the bed of the cyst and incorporated as part of the specimen. Terminal branches of the long sphenopalatine nerve are often seen in the capsule of the cyst. Identification of cholesterol in nasopalatine cysts is uncommon. The viscous fluid content may be mucoid material or pus if it has been infected.

Treatment

When there is irrefutable clinical evidence of an incisive canal cyst with or without abnormal radiographic enlargement of the fossa, treatment should be instituted. An incision is made around the gingival margins of the standing teeth or along the crest of the ridge in the edentulous patient. The size of the flap is governed by the posterior extent of the cyst and the required visual and mechanical access. For a small cyst the palatal flap raised should extend from canine to canine. It may be necessary to release the cyst from an attachment to the overlying mucoperiosteum with a knife, as this tissue structure is retracted. The neurovascular bundle is severed flush with the surface of the palatal bone and sufficient bone is removed to enable the upward extension of the cyst to be traced and freed. Careful dissection is necessary to detach the cyst from the bony cavity. The lining is often adherent to and continuous with the contents of the incisive canals above and the connection may need division with knife or scissors. Following enucleation blood clot is allowed to fill the empty cavity and a space filler is not inserted. In view of the slow progress of bone regeneration, which may be retarded by failure of periosteal reapposition, some operators advise the use of bone chips in an endeavour to obtain early obliteration of the defect. The flap is returned to its original position and the wound is closed by interrupted sutures taken through the interproximal spaces.

Cyst of the papilla palatina

Described as a distinct entity by Thoma and Brackett (1936), this cyst is alleged to develop either from epithelial contents of the incisive fossa or epithelium at the posterior border of the papilla. The mucosal covering at the papilla is normal but periodically a superficial, fluctuant, bluish swelling appears just behind it and then ruptures spontaneously with the discharge of a salty fluid. X-ray findings are negative. It is conceivable that this cystic formation is inaccurately designated, and that it represents merely an incisive canal cyst arising at the oral end of the intrabony passageway, but too small in diameter to be recognized radiographically. Removal of the cyst is best effected by excision of a small ellipse of palatal mucosa, circumscribing the area. The adjacent mucoperiosteum is raised and the wound closed with suture. If the edges cannot be approximated a small pack of gauze, soaked in Whitehead's varnish, is sutured in.

Nasolabial cyst

In describing these cysts the following alternative designations have been used: nasoalveolar cyst, nasoextra-alveolar cyst, nasal vestibule cyst, mucoid cyst of the nose, facial cleft or Klestadt cyst, nasal wing cyst, Gerber cyst and mucoid threshold cyst of the floor of the nose. The condition is uncommon, but Schroff (1929) reviewed 60 cases from the literature, Miller and Moore (1949) studied 82 cases, Montreuil (1949) collected 117 cases and Roed-Petersen (1969) 155 patients and quotes 97 papers. However, such series usually include only a small number of personal cases. Although the nasolabial cyst is strictly a soft tissue lesion, its inclusion with the fissural cyst of the jaws is a convenient and time-honoured practice.

The origin of nasolabial cysts has been the subject of considerable speculation and the views of various authors are reviewed by Seward (1962) and Roed-Petersen (1969). Lucas (1964) puts the origin at the junction of the globular, lateral nasal and maxillary processes. Sequestered epithelium from the depths of the nasomaxillary groove, which lies between the maxillary and lateral nasal processes, would seem to us to be the most likely source of the epithelial rests from which nasolabial cysts develop.

The majority of cases have been reported in adults, but Mathis (1957) quotes a case treated by Bartuals of a girl of 18 years of age who was said to have had the condition since childhood. Blumenthal (1913) describes a child aged 12 with such a cyst. Mostly, a single cyst is found on one side only, but bilateral cases have been reported. Roed-Petersen (1969) records 13 such patients of which two were his own. Schmidt (1931) comments that in bilateral cases the upper jaw forms a protruding bony septum between the two lesions, and Terracol (1936) states that the swelling gives the patient a mongoloid appearance.

Clinical findings

The lesion produces a visible external swelling of the lip, raises the alar cartilage, distorts the shape of the nose and the external nares and obliterates the nasolabial fold. An upwards extension into the nasal vestibule may eventually reach the inferior concha and thus interfere with breathing. In this situation the cyst is covered only by nasal mucous membrane, and occasionally it may rupture spontaneously into the nose, whereupon the swelling will disappear temporarily. Protrusion downwards between the lip and alveolar process will enable the lower border of the cyst to be palpated in the labial vestibule. Compression of the swelling in the sulcus will lead to enlargement of the one in the nasal vestibule. When an examining finger is inserted into the nostril and another into the buccal sulcus the extent of the lesion can be verified and fluctuation may be detected. If the flange of a denture bears upon it a denture granuloma will be produced which may disguise the nature of the swelling. The swelling is generally painless unless it becomes secondarily infected, and if this occurs there may be a sudden increase in size followed by a discharge of pus either from the nose or mouth. Sometimes a pain is reported which radiates to the infraorbital margin. This may be due to resorption of bone reaching the anterior superior dental neurovascular bundle.

Radiological examination

Many authors attach little importance to this investigation in the diagnosis of nasolabial cyst. It has been stated that because the lesion is separated from bone by periosteum, radiographic changes would be expected only if the enlargement had been present for a considerable period. However, it is incontrovertible that occasionally the cyst may cause pressure resorption of the underlying bone as in the case described by Hitchin (1946), and this may be demonstrated radiographically. Hermann (1932) recognized that the characteristic S-shaped bony border of the nasal entrance may show variations in contour as a result of resorption of the nasal notch. Seward (1962) stresses the differential diagnostic features which separate this cyst from others simulating it. In particular he describes the appearance seen in the standard occlusal view. In the normal patient the inferior margin of the anterior bony aperture of the nose, together with the buttress of the anterior nasal spine, form a bracket-shaped linear image. When the inferior margin is distorted by a nasolabial cyst a marked posterior convexity (backwards bowing) is produced in half of the bracket-shaped line. Hitchin (1962) has affirmed the diagnostic value of this observation, and he also shows how the shadow of the soft tissue swelling can be seen beneath the shadow of the distended upper lip in some cases. The shape and size of the cyst can be demonstrated radiographically by the injection of a radio-opaque substance such as Hypaque (Figs. 9.6, 9.7). Miller and Moore (1949), Boone (1955), Mathis (1957), Thoma and Goldman (1960), Seward (1962) and Roed-Petersen (1969), among others, have used contrast radiography.

Differential diagnosis

The infected nasolabial cyst might be confused with an acute alveolar abscess arising from an upper anterior tooth, and pulp tests of the adjoining maxillary incisors and canine should be carried out to avoid this error. It also should be differentiated from a nasal furuncle. Where the flange of a denture has induced a denture granuloma the presence of the underlying cyst might be overlooked, and either a large mucous extravasation cyst or a cystic salivary adenoma arising from an upper labial minor salivary gland could be mistaken for an uninfected nasolabial cyst.

E

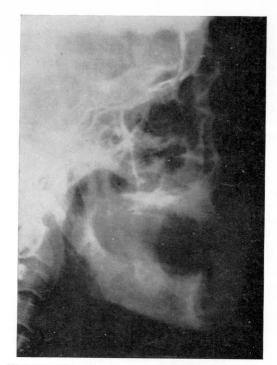

Fig. 9.6

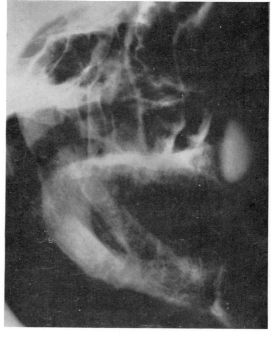

Fig. 9.7

Treatment

Nasolabial cysts are treated by excision under either general or local anaesthesia. An incision is made over the convexity of the swelling in the upper buccal sulcus. Incisions through the full thickness of the ridge mucoperiosteum are to be avoided because they open the wrong tissue plane, as the cyst lies extraperiosteally. The soft tissues are retracted and progressively dissected away from the cyst wall. There is often a firm adherence of the cyst to the cartilage of the ala and to the mucosa of the floor of the nose, and extra care will be needed at these sites. Should the mucosa of the nasal floor be perforated it should be mobilized for a short distance around the opening and closed with a few fine catgut sutures. Finally, the incision in the sulcus is closed with interrupted sutures, and a pressure dressing applied to the cheek for 24 hours to prevent a haematoma forming in the wound.

Pathological examination

Zuckerkandl (1882), giving what is considered to be the first clinical description, described the fluid as 'honey-like'. Often the fluid is referred to as straw-coloured and mucinous. Other times the contents are said to be whitish, glairy or mucoid. Many have stressed the absence of cholesterol crystals. The connective tissue capsule is lined by a pseudostratified columnar epithelium, or a cuboidal epithelium, both of which usually contain mucus-secreting goblet cells and are ciliated. A few are lined by stratified squamous epithelium and linings composed of all of these types are not uncommon (Boone 1955, Atterbury *et al.* 1961, Roed-Petersen 1969).

REFERENCES

Abrahams, A. M., Howell, F. V. & Bullock, W. K. (1963) *Oral Surg.,* **16,** 306.
Albers, D. D. (1973) *Oral Surg.,* **16,** 306.
Atterbury, R. A. Vazirani, S. J. & McNabb, W. J. (1961) *Oral Surg.,* **14,** 769.
Blumenthal, A. (1913) *Zeitschrift für Ohrenkeilkunde,* **68,** 60.
Boone, C. G. (1955) *Oral Surg.,* **8,** 40.
Hermann, M. (1932) Quoted by Holth, O. (1939) *Norkse Tunnlaege forenings Tidende,* **43,** 315.
Hitchin, A. D. (1946) *Brit. Dent. J.,* **80,** 53.
Hitchin, A. D. (1962) *Dent. Pract.,* 12, 252.
Hyde, W. H. (1942) *Dent. Items,* **64,** 105.
Lucas, R. B. (1964) *Pathology of Tumours of the Oral Tissues.* London: Churchill.
Lucchesi, F. J. & Topazian, D. S. (1961) *J. Oral Surg.,* **19,** 336.
Mathis, H. (1957), *Deutsche Zahnarztliche Zeitschrift,* **11,** 789.
Meyer, A. W. (1931) *Anat. Rec.* **49,** 19.

Figs. 9.6 and 9.7 True lateral radiographs of a West Indian patient who presented with a cystic swelling in the labial sulcus above /3. At its nasal end the swelling had protruded into the left nostril and occluded the air passage. The radiograph in Fig. 9.6 shows that the cyst was at first not demonstrable radiologically, but following the injection of a radio-opaque fluid the position and extent of the cyst could be determined. Histological examination confirmed the clinical diagnosis of a nasolabial cyst.

118 BENIGN CYSTIC LESIONS OF THE JAWS

Meyer, I. (1957) *Oral Surg.*, **10**, 175.
Miller, J. B., & Moore, P. M. (1949) *Annals of Otol., Rhinol. & Laryngol.*, **58**, 20.
Montreuil, F. (1949) *Annals of Otol., Rhinol. & Laryngol.*, **58**, 21.
Olech, E. (1957) *Oral Surg.*, **10**, 6.
Roed-Petersen, B. (1969) *Brit. J. Oral Surg.*, **7**, 84.
Roper-Hall, H. T. (1938) *Brit. Dent. J.*, **65**, 405.
Schroff, J. (1929) *Dent. Items*, **51**, 107.
Schmidt, J. (1931) *Deutsche Monatsschrift für zahnheilkunde*, **81**, 50.
Seward, G. R. (1956) *Dent. Practit.*, **6**, 212.
Seward, G. R. (1962) *Dental Practit.*, **12**, 154.
Seward, G. R. (1964) *Radiology in General Dental Practice*. London: British Dental Association.
Stafne, E. C. (1958) *Oral Roentgenographic Diagnosis*. Philadelphia: Saunders.
Terracol, J. (1936) *Maladies des Fosses Nasales*. Paris: Masson.
Thoma, K. H. & Brackett, C. A. (1936) *Int. J. Orthod. Dent. Child.*, **22**, 521.
Thoma, K. H. & Goldman, H. M. (1960) *Oral Pathology*. St. Louis: Mosby.
Zuckerkandl, E. (1882) *Normale und Pathologische Anatomie der Nasenhohle*. **1**, 85. Wien: Braumüller.

10. Bone Cysts

Solitary bone cyst

The solitary bone cyst has also been termed extravasation cyst, haemorrhagic bone cyst, traumatic bone cyst, simple bone cyst, unicameral cyst and progressive bone cavity. There has been controversy about the use of the word 'cyst' to describe this lesion when, in fact, the cavity does not have a microscopically demonstrable epithelial lining and it is even said, on occasions, to be devoid of a liquid content. However, an epithelial component is not essential for a fluid-filled cavity to be classified as a cyst. It is true that most cysts of the jaws are lined by epithelium, but many cysts elsewhere in the body have a lining which is devoid of epithelium. The designations 'extravasation', 'traumatic' and 'haemorrhagic' bone cysts were introduced to denote the origin of these cavities, but their aetiology is, in fact, still obscure and the more noncommittal titles are best used. Whinery (1955) suggested the name 'progressive bony cavity' to indicate its tendency to increase in size, but this assumption has not found general acceptance, because after initial steady enlargement growth is retarded and may cease altogether, with eventual spontaneous regression of a proportion of these defects.

The majority of bone cysts are located in the mandible between the canine and the third molar, although occasionally a lesion may develop in the incisor region or in the ramus of the mandible. The maxilla is rarely affected; for example, Gardner *et al.* (1962) observed only two bone cysts in the upper jaw in a review of 45 cases.

The occurrence of bony abnormalities of this type is not confined to the jaws, and similar cyst-like lesions are seen elsewhere in the skeleton with principal distribution at the proximal ends of the humerus and upper and lower portions of the femoral and tibial shafts, where they are known as unicameral cysts (Lodwick 1958). Jaffe and Lichtenstein (1942) maintain that some two-thirds of all such lesions occur in the humerus or femur. Cysts have been described in the humerus, femur, tibia, calcaneum, radius, fibula, ilium, ulnar, ribs and talus (Ogden and Griswold 1972). It is exceptional for more than one cyst to be found in the same patient (Boseker *et al.* 1968), but Hankey records a case in which three solitary bone cysts occurred in the mandible (Hankey 1947).

Clinical findings

The solitary bone cyst is usually symptomless, and it is frequently discovered fortuitously on routine radiography. Although the size attained may be considerable, bony enlargement at the expense of the cortical plates is less marked than with most other cysts of the jaws, although instances of marked expansion have been reported. The references to an expansile type include a paper by Fordyce (1964) who suggested that these lesions may account for 25 per cent of recorded cases. In our own series of 23 cases, 5 caused expansion of the jaw. In some instances in the molar region of the mandible the expansion is found on the lingual aspect, below the mylohyoid ridge, and may be overlooked unless specially angulated occlusal radiographs are taken. According to Olech *et al.* (1951, 1953, 1955) a bluish sheen may be visible on reflecting the mucoperiosteum overlying the defect, and as in the case of other cysts this is stated to be due to the translucency of the attenuated cortex.

In the mandible the neurovascular bundle may be freely exposed within the cavity, and it is logical to assume that labial anaesthesia would result if the cyst became acutely infected and filled with pus. Bennett and Chilton (1945) reported that encroachment upon the inferior dental canal might cause pain and labial anaesthesia, but in the authors' experience this view has not been substantiated. Sharma (1967), however, reports a case with a mild degree of paraesthesia of the lower lip which disappeared two months after a cyst in the lower premolar region had been operated upon. The teeth associated with the cyst retain their vitality and are not often loosened, despite extensions of the cyst into the interdental and interradicular bone. Of two large cysts described by Fordyce (1964), one displaced the unerupted third molar and prevented its eruption, the second did not and the third molar erupted normally.

Cysts are observed most frequently during the first or second decades. Fordyce (1964) states that he has been unable to find records of such a cyst in a patient over the age of 35 years. The ages of the patients seen by us have ranged widely; the oldest was 61 and three were aged more than 35 years. Nevertheless, these figures represent the age on detection, and do not imply that the cyst began its development then. The relatively infrequent solitary bone cysts in the older age groups might support the theory that the cavities eventually tend to undergo a natural cure. Three bony cavities followed radiologically by the authors eventually disappeared. In view of the manner in which the mere stimulation of bleeding into the defect can cause rapid healing, it is possible that spontaneous resolution of the cyst may be brought about by simple haemorrhage into the cavity following inadvertent trauma.

Radiological examination

Radiographically the cyst is variable in size and may extend from the body of the mandible into the ascending ramus. It appears as a unilocular cavity which is not trabeculated but which may exhibit ridges on its internal surface. In the premolar-molar region of the mandible the lesion may project upwards into the interradular septa, producing a scalloped contour around the roots of standing teeth (Fig. 10.1). The contour is regular

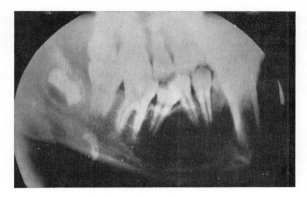

Fig. 10.1 Lateral oblique film of a solitary bone cyst showing the 'scalloping' effect between adjoining teeth.

in the anterior region and the general shape is round or oval with no indentations between the teeth. The growing edge of the lesion never seems to perforate the alveolar crest even when the lesion is extensive. Roots of the adjacent teeth may be displaced but eventual realignment occurs after surgical exploration of the defect. Teeth whose roots are in immediate proximity to the cyst are not often resorbed, nor do the teeth become devitalized or mobile. Usually an intact lamina dura can be traced around the roots which invaginate the cyst cavity, but occasionally the lamina dura is partly destroyed. The periphery of the radiolucent area is clearly demarcated but often devoid of a circumferential white limiting line. Indeed, it is exceptional to see a white line about a cyst posterior to the lower canine, but not unusual to see such a line about one anterior to the canine. Although distension of the outer or inner plate is uncommon, when suspected an occlusal film should be taken.

Contents

On investigation, these cavities are often reported to be empty, but usually contain a golden-yellow fluid. Blood-stained fluid or clot, when present, indicates recent haemorrhage, perhaps even during the operation, because degradation of blood or phagocytosis and absorption of clot requires only a comparatively short time – not more than a week or two at the most. Indeed, if fluid is aspirated from such cysts for diagnostic purposes it must be done with considerable care, for the surrounding blood vessels are fragile and a fall in pressure within the cyst wall will induce bleeding.

Some authors report that these cysts are empty. Whether examples filled only with gas exist is difficult to say, since it would depend how carefully they were investigated. Often the operator is not expecting the cyst to be a solitary bone cyst but believes he is operating on a more commonly seen cyst of the jaws. After the cavity has been opened and all the blood aspirated away, the surgeon is able to observe that there is not a dissectable lining and describes the cavity as 'empty'. There seems to be little doubt that the fluid in these cysts is under less pressure than in others, and there is not the gush of liquid, shimmering with cholesterol, that flows from a radicular or dentigerous cyst. Neither is there the creamy white liquid which escapes from a keratocyst. Thus, unless special precautions are taken, any contained liquid can escape detection. Moreover, there is no lining epithelium, but if the cavity is gently washed out and inspected, a delicate smooth membrane of connective tissue may be seen like a sheen on the walls. Indeed, if the cyst extends into the alveolar process and can be transilluminated, blood vessels (as in the web of a frog's foot) are seen coursing over the wall. Tenuous folds of soft tissue will run to the apices of any roots protruding into the cavity and contain their apical nerves and vessels in the free edge. Pinkish gelatinous masses may be found adherent to the recesses in the wall. These are composed of foam cells and may represent blood clot which is being removed. The cavity wall is not smooth but has a craggy, unfinished appearance, and it is easy to induce bleeding from the bone.

Since the cavity of a solitary bone cyst is most unlikely to contain a vacuum but is devoid of soft tissue, and regularly reputed to be empty of liquid, it is interesting to speculate upon a possible gaseous content. It is improbable that either oxygen or carbon dioxide is present, and a plausible theory is that nitrogen diffuses into the space. Gas-filled cysts within the wall of the large bowel are a recognized entity, but their contents are unknown. It has been shown that the liquid in unicameral cysts of long bones often contains a yellow-coloured fluid (Cohen 1960). Seward (1963) reported similarly that the fluid in mandibular cysts is, in his experience, golden yellow in colour, clots on standing and contains a high concentration of bilirubin. Further observations since then have confirmed this. Special care must be taken during recovery of the fluid. A flap is reflected and the overlying bone surface dried. If it is thick, it may be drilled but not perforated, with a rosehead bur. A wide-bore needle on a syringe is pushed in and a much smaller one introduced alongside. A Toller double-lumen aspirating needle is ideal. The opposite wall should not be struck by the needle point, and a small quantity of liquid only is aspirated. An attempt should not be made to aspirate the cavity dry or bleeding will be induced. The presence of bilirubin suggests previous haemorrhage into the cavity and, moreover, that the pigment is unable to escape into lymphatics as is its usual fate. Examples of solitary bone cyst fluids are given in Table 10.1.

Pathological examination

On microscopical examination the bony walls are found to be covered by a delicate layer of loose connective tissue containing congested capillary vessels, extravasated red blood cells, haemosiderin pigment and multinucleated giant cells. The adjoining bone shows evidence of lacunar

Table 10.1 Fluid analysis from solitary bone cysts

Sex	Age (years)	Total plasma protein (mg 100 ml)	Albumin (mg per cent)	Globulin (mg per cent)	Electrophoresis	Bilirubin Content (mg/100 ml)
Female	30	7.6	5.2	2.9	Normal strip	2.0
Male	15	5.5	3.7	1.8	Reduced $_2$ globulin	4.3
*Female	26	6.3	4.6	1.7	Normal strip	2.4
Female	12	6	3.7	2.3	Normal strip	8.6

*Chloride 100 mmol/1, sodium 142 mmol/1, potassium 5.2 mmol/1–shows a low potassium compared with serum.

resorption but only at intervals. At other sites there is inactivity, or even bone deposition suggesting intermittent and slow enlargement of the cavity. New bone is deposited subperiosteally and this is usually lamellar bone; again implying only slow enlargement. Occasionally woven bone is found subperiosteally or even on the cavity aspect. It is clear from the histological appearance that the balance between healing and progression is a fine one, and that it is compatible with the view that spontaneous healing can occur.

Differential diagnosis

The differential diagnosis of solitary bone cyst from other cysts of the jaws is simplified by aspiration, for it is the only type which has a fluid containing marked concentrations of bilirubin. Radiographically it may be difficult to distinguish between solitary bone cysts and primordial (kerato) cysts, but aspiration will readily distinguish between the two as their liquid contents are quite different.

Other similar radiographical appearances are disuse atrophy and Gaucher's disease. The latter should present no problem since the other general signs of the disease, enlarged liver and spleen etc. will be present. Further aspiration may recover typical Gaucher's cells from the marrow. Disuse atrophy usually can be distinguished by considering the loss of teeth and pattern of stress on the jaw. Persistent zones of red bone marrow in older subjects where the marrow is normally fatty may be contained in discrete medullary compartments, devoid of trabecular bone. Attention was drawn to these by Standish and Shafer (1962). These zones can be quite difficult to distinguish from a small bone cyst and a period of observation may be required. It has been suggested that some supposed bone cysts which have 'healed' spontaneously represent such zones of red marrow which subsequently have been replaced by fatty marrow and have been penetrated by bony trabeculae. Another possible point of difficulty is the medullary cavity in the lower premolar region.

Here it is not unusual for trabeculae of bone to be scanty or absent and a marked form of this normal anatomical appearance may suggest a solitary bone cyst.

Complications

The only possible complication of solitary bone cysts is pathological fracture. This seems to be an uncommon occurrence for bone cysts in the jaws, but Sieverink (1974) records such a case (his Case 5). According to Garceau and Gregory (1954), 65 per cent of long bone lesions are discovered in this way, and they record a case in which non-union resulted.

Treatment

Surgical exploration of the area should be carried out to confirm the diagnosis. This also constitutes the treatment, for it has been found that opening such cysts, evacuating the contents and making them bleed results in rapid obliteration of the defect with new bone. Space-filling material such as bone chips is not required. The practical advantages of surgical intervention are restoration of the normal architecture of the jaw and elimination of a potential site for pathological fracture. Blum (1955) considered that many cases healed spontaneously and this may be so. However, if there is no exploration there is no definitive diagnosis, and the clinician would need care and some courage in advocating such a course of action. Fordyce (1964) did observe a case in the hope of regression, because the parents were against surgery, but exploration was eventually necessary. Others, e.g. Biewald (1967), advocate aspiration and the injection of autogenous venous blood. There are rare occasions when this alone is justifiable and, in the authors' experience, can be successful, but such cases must be followed with due care.

Following surgical exploration the majority of bone cysts of the jaws heal rapidly. Vijayaraghaven and Whitlock (1975) record a case which recurred twice following exploration and packing. However, at age 19, the cavity started to fill in with bone. The mandible was contoured to the shape of the other side and full healing occurred. Perhaps it is noteworthy that this case was first treated at the age of 7½ years, whereas most cases are discovered and treated during the second decade or later.

Indeed, the behaviour of the jaw cyst in this case is not unlike that of the long bone cysts, some one-third of which recur even when they have been filled with bone chips. It is notable, however, that the long bone cysts are often found and treated during the first decade.

Comment. The origin of the solitary bone cyst is still in doubt, but a number of theories as to its causation have been advanced. A widely held view is the traumatic-haemorrhagic theory advanced by Pommer in 1920. This postulates that haemorrhage occurs in the bone as a result of injury, and then failure of organization and subsequent liquefaction of the clot ensues. The advocates of this' theory suggest that a barrier of necrotic elements forms between the surrounding vital tissue and the blood clot, preventing the establishment of an active blood circulation which is necessary for normal organization. When gradual increase in the dimensions of the lesions takes place, it is postulated that the transudation of fluid into the space produced by the unresolved haematoma causes in turn a pressure resorption of the surrounding bone and possible expansion of the overlying cortical plate. It is further explained that healing is prevented by the encapsulated haematoma, but that normal remodelling activity proceeds along the circumference of the bony defect. What is not explained is how the necrotic medullary trabeculae are removed from the centre of the haematoma. If this theory is correct, solitary bone cysts should be common following jaw fractures. This is not the case, and Pommer suggests that when the periosteum is torn as in fractures the possibility of the closed pressure effect is nullified. Another difficulty is acceptance of the concept of a haemorrhage into the medulla of a normal mandible without sufficient distortion of the bone occurring to cause a fracture. The fact that on direct questioning most patients with a solitary bone cyst can recall having suffered a blow on the jaw means little, since everyone has sustained similar trauma on some occasion, yet the general incidence of solitary bone cysts amongst the population at large is infinitesimal. If these lesions are caused by trauma it should be anticipated that some damage to the teeth might also result, but a salient feature of these lesions is that the teeth remain vital and chipped incisors – so frequently a residue of trauma in childhood – are not seen.

In 1917, Bland Sutton suggested that the solitary bone cysts may arise as the result of spontaneous atrophy of the tissue of a central benign giant-cell lesion. One of the authors has followed for many years a patient who initially was under the care of G. T. Hankey and had a central giant-cell granuloma of the right mandibular molar region. This diagnosis was established by a generous biopsy. Following biopsy the lesion healed, but recurred three years later. The new lesion, similar in appearance radiographically and at the same site, was explored and a solitary bone cyst discovered. This in turn healed to leave an enlarged side to the mandible with a radiographic appearance resembling fibrous dysplasia of bone. Small spherical cavities appeared and disappeared in this bone spontaneously. Slow remodelling followed, but ten years elapsed before the normal contour of the jaw was restored.

On the other hand, most giant-cell granulomas are found a decade later or more than is common for solitary bone cysts so a frequent relationship is unlikely.

Another hypothesis is that they are caused by an upset in calcium metabolism (Whinery 1955), but relevant blood chemistry investigations are always within the range of normal. The interesting explanation that a low-grade osteomyelitis is responsible for the condition stems from Phemister and Gordon (1926) but there is no real evidence to support this contention.

After considering the natural history of personal cases and the problem of reconciling the phenomenon of spontaneous regression of some lesions, it is possible that some upset of the normal physiological process of bone reconstruction may be the mechanism responsible for the formation and perpetuation of the cyst (Killey and Kay 1964).

Geschickter and Copeland (1949) suggested this for the long bone lesions. They proposed an excessive continuation of the remodelling resorption at the metaphyseal-epiphyseal junction region. In the long bones it is in this region where the cysts start to appear and it has been noted that their growth is often arrested when they move further into the shaft with an increase in length of the bone. Moreover, the closer the cyst is to the epiphyseal region, the more likely it is to recur after operation. While the authors have seen two solitary bone cysts in the ramus, one of which intruded into the condyle, no case has been reported in which there was enlargement of the condyle head only, suggesting an origin close to the growth cartilage. On the other hand, this is not a site of marked remodelling resorption as in the long bones.

Many bone and joint lesions are attributable to decompression sickness in compressed air workers. The lesions resulting from this avascular or aseptic necrosis consist of sclerotic changes in the medulla, which often terminate as 'lakes' in the bone, and a varying degree of destruction of the articular surfaces (Golding et al. 1960). It has been suggested that the pathogenesis of destructive changes in the long bones from decompression is due to nitrogen emboli in the nutrient vessels or gas formation in the medullary fat. If the articular surface is involved painful symptoms arise, but those lesions in the shaft are clinically silent (McCallum et al. 1954). Such infarcts may produce a cyst-like lesion of the medullary bone which is devoid of contents or contains only a small quantity of fluid which does not fill the cavity. The cysts are symptomless, and can be cured by making them bleed since this is followed by invasion of new bone. Occasionally spontaneous regeneration occurs without surgical interference – the radiolucent area in the medullary bone disappears and the bone becomes radiologically normal. Thus these cyst-like cavities in medullary bone, resulting either from infarction caused by nitrogen emboli or compression of the vascular supply by nitrogen bubbles, bear an interesting resemblance to the solitary bone cyst of the jaws.

Similar lesions are sometimes seen in patients who have never worked in compressed air, but these are less likely to be multiple. Fat embolism, bland infarcts or arteriosclerosis of nutrient vessels have all been suggested as the possible cause (Kahlstrom 1942, Taylor 1944). Jones and Sakovich (1966) have shown by animal experimentation that it is possible to occlude intraosseous capillaries with lipiodol fat emboli which are detectable in their impacted positions at least five weeks after infusion.

Avascular necrosis in the head of a long bone may also develop following long-term corticosteroid therapy (Epstein et al. 1965); and similar ischaemia may be produced by terminal vessel thrombosis in such condition as lupus erythematosus, rheumatoid arthritis, haemophilia, Gaucher's disease, sickle-cell anaemia and congenital haemolytic anaemia. Bone cysts similar to solitary bone cysts may be found in patients with hyperparathyroidism, but they are usually small and should not be confused with the so-called radiographic 'cysts' which are usually known as 'brown nodes' and happen to be solid lesions.

Toller (1964) was able to make a number of interesting and original observations on a case, the clinical features of which were described by Fordyce (1964). The hydrostatic pressure within the cyst was measured by a sensitive manometer and recorded as 5 cm of water. This is exceptionally low compared with epithelium-lined cysts and comparable with capillary pressure. A golden fluid not contaminated by recent haemorrhage was aspirated (we would expect such a fluid to contain a high concentration of bilirubin). The protein content was similar to serum, except that the alpha globulin was reduced in quantity on a paper electrophoretogram. The osmotic tension of the cyst fluid was greater than that of the patient's blood, but the pressure difference was lower than capillary pressure. This explained how the capillaries in the delicate connective tissue lining remained patent.

The cyst wall acted as a semipermeable membrane and the radioactive substances introduced were not cleared into the lymphatics or blood system. There was, therefore, no lymphatic access to the cyst cavity. Induced haemorrhage appeared to produce a temporary marked rise in intracystic pressure.

In a paper to the Royal Society of Medicine Section of Odontology, Soskolne (1972) made observations on the pathogenesis and morphology of giant-cell granulomas of the jaws. He examined the thin-walled, dilated vessels in these lesions, some of which contained varying numbers of red blood corpuscles and an eosinophilic, homogeneous material, and he stated that they were identical, ultrastructurally, to lymphatic vessels. On the other hand they could be sinusoidal blood vessels of a simple structure, for it is reputed that lymphatic channels do not occur in the bone marrow.

A view on the genesis of these cysts can be put forward which brings together a number of these various opinions. The presence of bilirubin in the fluid is both evidence for past haemorrhage into the cysts and a lack of a pathway for the fluid out into the lymphatics. If 'lymphatics' like those found by Soskolne in giant-cell granulomas or similar endothelium-lined vascular channels were to be present normally, or in some pre-existing lesion, it is conceivable that they could become cut off from the normal circulation. It is possible that abnormal sinusoids might develop without a connection to the circulation. Under the circumstances fluid would tend to enter the sinusoid, but could not escape either into the circulation or into the lymphatics and would dilate. Gitlin (1955) points out that where there is an obstruction to lymphatic flow, the concentration of proteins of the enclosed fluid approximates to that of serum. Such a dilated sinusoid would be like an intrabony cystic hygroma.

Toller has noted changes in pressure (or volume) as measured by his manometer within the cyst with swallowing movements. These perhaps reflect venous engorgement of the small vessels in the cyst wall. More violent interruption of respiratory movements like coughing or sneezing might therefore induce capillary bleeding into the cyst. Possibly, alterations in stress upon the mandible or a blow might similarly induce haemorrhage with a temporary increase in the internal pressure. Variations in internal pressure following such small haemorrhages might account for the phasic enlargement and healing of such cysts. If one were to postulate some other factor which altered the balance between enlargement and healing and which occurred in early adult life, together with a larger than average haemorrhage, then complete healing might follow as when autogenous blood is injected.

Statistical analysis

A provisional diagnosis of solitary bone cyst was made following clinical and radiological examination of 23 cyst-like lesions in the mandible. The diagnosis was confirmed by operation in 17 cases. Four patients declined surgical intervention on the grounds that the lesion was causing them no inconvenience, and follow-up radiographs over a period of years have shown a spontaneous regeneration of bone within each defect with eventual disappearance of the radiolucent area. For specific reasons two suspected solitary bone cysts have not been explored surgically, but the patients are being reviewed at regular intervals. Details of the entire group of 23 cases appear in Table 10.2.

With regard to the 17 patients whose lesions were investigated surgically, the ages ranged from 11 to 61 years. Of these, 12 individuals were under the age of 23 years and with two exceptions were either adolescents or young adults. In two of the three cases of spontaneous regression the patients concerned were also adolescents, and the remaining two patients who were not operated upon were in the teenage group. This predominance in incidence of occurrence with respect to the second decade of life conforms with the experience of previous observers.

The sex distribution for the 17 established cases showed a small preponderance of affected females (8:6). Of the three cases in which natural healing took place two were in females. The two unoperated patients were of opposite sex.

On examination of the complete case list no lesions were located in the maxilla, and in the lower jaw the site of predilection was the premolar-molar region. Only three solitary bone cysts were positioned anterior to the canine, and all of these cavities had a regular shape with no lobulation of their margins.

Expansion was detected in six of the 17 proved cases, which represents an approximate incidence of one in every three. Spontaneous regression

Table 10.2 Solitary bone cysts

Case no.	Age	Sex	Site	Size (diameter in cm)	Shape	Vitality of related tooth	Expansion	Labial anaesthesia	Cavity contents	Pathological Examination	Blood chemistry (serum calcium, phosphorus and alkaline phosphatase	Final radiological result
1	17	F	87/	2.5 x 1.5	Ovoid with regular margin	Vital	Nil	Nil	Not explored. Declined operation		Normal	Spontaneous. Regression achieved in 3 years
2	20	F	7654/	5 x 2	Ovoid with scalloped margin	Vital	Lingual and buccal (slight)	Nil	Pieces of fibrous tissue. No fluid	Fibrous tissue layer	Normal	Healing satisfactorily but failed follow-up
3	17	F	321/123	3.5 x 1.5	Ovoid with scalloped margin	Vital	Buccal (slight)	Nil	Straw-coloured fluid		Not performed	Healed completely in 1½ years
4	21	M	/567	4 x 2	Ovoid with scalloped margin	Vital	Nil	Nil	Empty		Not performed	Partial obliteration of defect in 8 months
5	11	F	543/	4 x 1.5	Pseudo-loculated	Vital	Buccal (slight)	Nil	Empty		Normal	Healed completely in 1 year
6	17	M	8765/	5 x 2	Ovoid with scalloped margin	Vital	Nil	Nil	Empty			Partial obliteration of defect in 9 months
7	15	M	321/123	2.5 x 2.5	Circular	Vital	Nil	Nil	Fibrous tissue	Shreds of fibrous tissue containing cells resembling lymphocytes. Specimen contains small areas of dysplastic coarse-fibred bone	Not performed	Healed completely in 1 year
8	39	F	/45678	8.5 x 1.5	Sausage-shaped	Vital	Nil	Nil	Empty		Not performed	Healed completely in 15 months
9	61	F	/678	7.5 x 2.5	Ovoid with regular margin	Edentulous	Nil	Nil	No lining or fluid but some dry crystals		Not performed	Healed completely in 1½ years

continued overleaf

Table 10.2 Solitary bone cysts — continued

Case no.	Age	Sex	Site	Size (diameter in cm)	Shape	Vitality of related tooth	Expansion	Labial anaesthesia	Cavity contents	Pathological Examination	Blood chemistry (serum calcium, phosphorus and alkaline phosphatase	Final radiological result
10	38	F	87/	1.5 x 1.5	Circular with regular margin	Vital	Nil	Nil	Not explored Declined operation		Normal	Spontaneous regression achieved in 2½ years
11	18	F	/78	2 x 1.5	Ovoid with regular margin	Vital	Nil	Nil	Not explored		Normal	Under review
12	17	M	/567	2 x 1.5	Ovoid with regular margin	Vital	Nil	Nil	Not explored		Normal	Under review
13	56	M	/4567	4 x 3	Ovoid	Edentulous	Buccal (slight)	Nil	Fibrous tissue	Specimen consists of fragments of vital lamellar bone surrounded by connective tissue, some areas of which are chronically inflamed	Not performed	Healed completely in 1½ years
14	20	F	/1234	2.5 x 2	Ovoid	Vital	Nil	Nil	Fibrous tissue and serosanguinous fluid	Young fibrous tissue containing trabeculae of newly formed woven bone and small amount of dysplastic ostcoid. No epithelial lining	Not performed	Healed completely in 15 months
15	14	M	/345	3.5 x 2	Ovoid	Vital	Nil	Nil	Not explored. Declined operation		Not performed	Spontaneous regression achieved in 3 years.
16	15	M	543/	1.5 x 1	Ovoid	Vital	Nil	Nil	Empty		Normal	Healed completely in 1½ years

Table 10.2 Solitary bone cysts – continued

Case no.	Age	Sex	Site	Size (diameter in cm)	Shape	Vitality of related tooth	Expansion	Labial anaesthesia	Cavity contents	Pathological Examination	Blood chemistry (serum calcium, phosphorus and alkaline phosphatase)	Final radiological result
17	43	M	765/	2.5 x 1.5	Ovoid	Edentulous	Nil	Nil	Fibrous tissue	Shreds of fibrous tissue. Trabeculae of woven bone cellular tissue containing multinucleated giant cells. Extravasated red blood cells and haemosiderin	Not performed	Partial regeneration in 8 months
18	22	F	8/	2 x 2	Circular with regular margin	Vital	Nil	Nil	Empty		Not performed	Healed completely in 1 year
19	30	F	/56	2 x 1.5	Ovoid with regular margin	Vital	Buccal (slight)	Nil	Empty		Normal	Partial regeneration in 1 year
20	11	F	Left ascending ramus	2.5	Ovoid	Vital	Nil	Nil	Empty	Shreds of fibrous tissue	Not performed	Healed
21	21	F	23456/	4	Scalloped between roots	Vital	Nil	Nil	Not explored. Declined operation		Not performed	Present without change 4 years
22	18	F	7/	2	Ovoid	Vital	Nil	Nil	Empty		Calcium 10.2 inorganic phosphorus 4.6, alkaline phosphatase 13	Healed in 1 year
23	25	M	/5	3 x 3	Ovoid	Vital	Nil	Nil	Small quantity of yellowish fluid	Thin layer of fibrous tissue	Not performed	Bone healing

occurred in three examples of the non-expansile type, which reinforces the view that if this form of solitary bone cyst were left untreated it would probably become obliterated by a natural process of bone re-formation. However, spontaneous regression in cases of the expansile variety is reputed to be unlikely.

In selected patients, diagnostic blood determinations of the levels of serum calcium, inorganic phosphorus and alkaline phosphatase were carried out. All values were within normal limits.

Those teeth related to solitary bone cysts in this series were vital preoperatively, and continued to give a normal response after surgical investigation of the cavity.

Aneurysmal bone cysts

The aneurysmal bone cyst was first described as a distinct clinical entity by Jaffe and Lichtenstein in 1942. Since then there have been additional examples of the condition recorded in the literature, and in 1957 Lichtenstein reported personal observations on 50 cases. In the past the lesion has been classified as an atypical giant-cell tumour or benign bone cyst.

The abnormality occurs mainly in children, adolescents or young adults, and there is no marked sex predominance. Cysts have been found in all parts of the skeleton but the vast majority occur in the spine and the long bones. Characteristically this benign solitary lesion causes local expansion, but the growth is non-infiltrative and a thin layer of overlying subperiosteal new bone is preserved in most cases. The lesion starts subperiosteally and initially produces a smooth, rounded soft tissue mass. At this stage it may be tender and either firm or springy. Incision is complicated by profuse bleeding. Subperiosteal new bone is laid down over the surface and resorption of the underlying cortex produces an eccentric cavity in the bone. Ridges on the walls of the cavity and septa of new bone may produce a soap-bubble appearance. The name 'aneurysmal bone cyst' derives from the 'blown out' appearance as seen in radiographs. In the long bone it starts in the metaphysis rather than the epiphysis. In the spine it can spread to involve several adjacent vertebrae. If untreated the cysts will increase in size gradually and become so large that amputation of a limb may be necessary or, if several vertebrae are involved, an irreversible paraplegia may result due to a pressure effect on the cord. Reports of lesions in the jaws are limited, but cases have been described by Bernier and Bhaskar (1958), Bhaskar et al. (1959), Wang (1960) and Vianna and Horizonte (1962). The paper presented by Bernier and Bhaskar concerned an 11-year-old girl and a 59-year-old woman; each patient presented with a swelling in the ramus region which radiographically showed as a unilocular radiolucent destructive lesion. The case Wang reported was that of an eight-year-old girl whose lesion was situated in the maxilla, as was the cyst described by Vianna.

Aetiology

The aetiology of these cysts is unknown. Many are said to be associated with a history of trauma but it is doubtful whether injury could initiate such a peculiar bone lesion. If the blood within the space is only the result of trauma this should lead to the formation of granulation tissue and callus (Donaldson 1962). A collateral suggestion made by Bernier and Bhaskar (1958) and other authorities is that the lesion in the jaws might represent a process analogous to the giant-cell reparative granuloma in which there is an exuberant attempt at repair of a haematoma. Reasons for rejecting such interpretations of the pathogenesis were detailed by Lichtenstein (1953).

In considering the second hypothesis of a possible relationship with the giant-cell lesion, it would have to be postulated that the haematoma maintains a circulatory connection with the damaged vessel. A slow flow of blood through the cyst could account for the clinical welling-up of blood when the lesion is operated upon.

A widely accepted theory is that the condition is caused by some variation in the haemodynamics or vascular supply of the area. Lichtenstein adheres to this view, for he stated in 1950 that the lesion might result from venous thrombosis or an arteriovenous aneurysm leading to increased venous pressure and the subsequent development of a dilated and engorged vascular bed in the bone area. It is assumed that resorption of bone by giant cells then occurs and this is replaced by connective tissue, osteoid and new bone.

Another aetiological concept is that the cyst is a secondary manifestation developing in a pre-existing lesion altered by haemorrhage, cystic degeneration or some other pathological process. However, it is evident from perusal of the literature that the factors concerned in the evolution of this complex pathological entity are still not clear and even Jaffe (1958) contends that the question of the origin and basic nature of the lesion still has to be left open. In our view it seems likely that this entity is a vascular giant cell granuloma.

Radiological examination

The jaw is often grossly expanded and outlined by an intact thin shell of bone which produces the typical ballooned-out appearance which Jaffe referred to as a 'subperiosteal blow-out'. Later the lesion may 'explode' with disintegration of the limiting cortical layer. The radiolucent area is either unilocular or multilocular, and may have a trabecular pattern which Worth (1963) described as a soap-bubble appearance.

Treatment

The lesion is amenable to treatment by curettage or local excision and this is the method of choice in a surgically accessible lesion. Jaffe recommends packing the cavity with autogenous bone chips following curettage. During the operation the surgeon may be hampered by persistent bleeding from the bed of the lesion. Radiotherapy has been used successfully and this provides an alternative when surgical extirpation is difficult, as in aneurysmal bone cysts of the vertebrae. Dosage within the range of 1400 to 2000 rads has been recommended by Wang, but Lichtenstein has reported a case where radiation sarcoma occurred after a latent period of many years following treatment of an aneurysmal bone cyst by irradiation. After healing of the wound, frequent post-operative radiographs are essential to demonstrate the progress of bone regeneration in the cyst cavity.

Recurrence of an aneurysmal bone cyst may occur following inadequate removal and a second operation will be required. According to Donaldson (1962) even incomplete eradication of the mass may produce a satisfactory result in some cases.

Pathological examination

Macroscopically when the mass is explored it is found to contain pools of venous blood and reddish-brown soft tissue which resembles a blood-filled sponge. Resultant bleeding is a persistent ooze which may be difficult to control, rather than a sudden spurting or vigorous free haemorrhage.

Microscopically, the area involved by the lesion is honeycombed by numerous intercommunicating vascular spaces which vary widely in size and are lined by flattened cells and filled with uncoagulated blood. The intervening septa consist of a cellular connective tissue, osteoid and immature bone permeated by foci of haemosiderin-containing macrophages and many giant cells of the foreign body type. In general the stroma resembles that of the giant-cell granuloma. However, it should be emphasized that the bone cavity is usually filled with the sponge-like soft tissue, so that the lesion is not really cystic.

REFERENCES

Bennett, I. B. & Chilton, N. W. (1945) *J. Am. Dent. Ass.,* **32,** 51.
Bernier, J. L. & Bhaskar, S. M. (1958) *J. Oral Surg.,* **11,** 1018.
Bhaskar, S. M., Bernier, J. L. & Godby, S. (1959) *J. Oral Surg.,* **17,** 30.
Biewald, H. F. (1967) *J. oral Surg.,* **25,** 427.
Bland-Sutton, J. (1917) *Tumours, Innocent and Malignant,* 6th ed. St Louis: Mosby
Blum, T. H. (1955) *Oral Surg.,* **8,** 917.
Boseker, E. H., Bickel, W. H. & Duhlin, D. C. (1968) *Surg. Gynec. & Obstet.,* **127,** 550.
Cohen, J. (1960) *J. Bone & Joint Surg.,* **42A,** 609.
Donaldson, W. F. (1962) *J. Bone Jt. Surg.,* **44A,** 25.
Epstein, N. N., Tuffonelli, D. L., & Epstein, J. H. (1965) *Archs. Derm.,* **92,** 178.
Fordyce, G. L. (1964) *Brit. J. Oral Surg.,* **2,** 80.
Garceau, G. J. & Gregory, R. F., (1954) *J. Bone & Joint Surg.,* **36A,** 267.
Gardner, A. F., Stoller, S. M. & Steig, H. M. (1962) *J. Canad. Dent. Ass.,* **28,** 151.
Geschickter, C. F. & Copeland, M. M. (1949) *Tumours of Bone,* 3rd ed. Philadelphia: Lippincott.
Gitlin, D. (1955) *Pediatrics,* **16,** 345.
Golding, F. C., Griffiths, P., Hempleman, H. V., Paton, W. D. & Walder, D. N. (1960) *Brit. J. Industr. Med.,* **17,** 167.

Hankey, G. T. (1947) Three cysts of the mandible, not of dental origin. *Proc. roy. Soc. Med.,* **40,** 723–726.
Jaffe, H. L. & Lichtenstein, L. (1942) *Arch. Surg.,* **44,** 1004.
Jones, J. P. & Sakovich, L. (1966) *J. Bone & Jt. Surg.,* **48A,** 149.
Kahlstrom, S. C. (1942) *Am. J. Roentg.,* **47,** 405.
Killey, H. C. & Kay, L. W. (1964) *J. Int. Coll. Surg.,* **42,** No. 5, 504.
Lichtenstein, C. (1957) *J. Bone Jt. Surg.,* **39A,** 873.
Lichtenstein, L. (1953) *Cancer,* **6,** 1228.
Lodwick, G. S. (1958) *Am. J. Roentg.,* **80,** 495.
McCallum, R. I. *et. al.* (1954) *J. Bone & Jt. Surg.,* **36B,** 606.
Ogden, J. A. & Griswold, D. M. (1972) *J. Bone & Joint Surg.,* **54A,** 1309.
Olech, E., Sicker, H. & Weinman, J. P. (1951) *Oral Surg.,* **4,** 1160.
Olech, E., Sicker, H. & Weinman, J. P. (1953) *Dent. Radiol. & Photog.,* **26,** 57.
Olech, E., Sicker, H. & Weinman, J. P. (1955) *Oral Surg.,* **8,** 962.
Phemister, D. B. & Gordon, J. E. (1926) *JAMA,* **87,** 1429.
Pommer, G. (1920) *Arch. Orth. Unfall-Chir,* **17,** 17.
Seward, G. R. (1963) *Brit. dent. J.,* **115,** 229.
Sharma, J. N. (1967) *Oral Surg.,* **24,** 211.
Sieverink, N. P. J. B. (1974) *The Single Bone Cyst,* p. 50. Nijmegen: Drukkery Schippers.
Soskolne, W. A. (1972) *Proc. roy. Soc. Med.,* **65,** 1131.
Standish, S. M. & Shafer, W. G. (1962) *J. Oral Surg.,* **20,** 123.
Taylor, H. K. (1944) *Radiology,* **42,** 550.
Toller, P. A. (1964) *Brit. J. Oral Surg.,* **2,** 86.
Vianna, M. R. & Horizonte, B. (1962) *J. oral Surg.,* **20,** 432.
Vijayaraghaven, K. & Whitlock, R. I. H. (1975) *Brit. J. Oral Surg.,* **13,** 64.
Wang, S. Y. (1960) *Plast. Reconstr. Surg.,* **25,** 62.
Whinery, J. G. (1955) *Oral Surg.,* **8,** 903.
Worth, H. M. (1963) *Principles and Practice of Oral Radiologic Interpretation.* Chicago: Year Book.

11. Multiple Cysts of the Jaws

The occurrence of multiple cysts of the jaw in an individual is rare. Most published cases have purported to be multiple dentigerous cysts. At the time at which they were reported a clear distinction was not made between multiple primary dentigerous cysts and multiple keratocysts. Maccaferri (1953) recorded bilateral dentigerous cysts in a boy of seven years of age, whilst Seeman (1937) described dentigerous cysts in all four quadrants of the mouth, and other cases have been observed by Oliver (1934), Bennett (1937), Ivy (1939), McGregor (1945), Sharland (1948) and Caldwell and Thompson (1955).

Multiple dentigerous cysts tend to be located in different quadrants of the mouth and are often present in both the upper and lower jaw, or they may arise symmetrically on both sides at about the time when, normally, the involved tooth would erupt (Figs. 11.1–11.3). They must be distinguished from the multiple dentigerous cysts which are keratocysts, many of which are extrafollicular in nature and which are part of the multiple cyst–basal cell naevus syndrome.

Most practitioners of some years' standing will have encountered

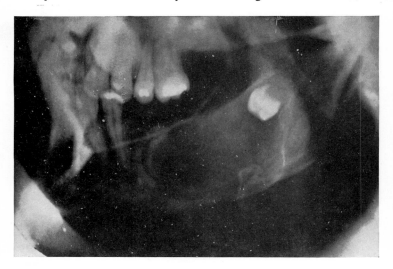

Fig. 11.1

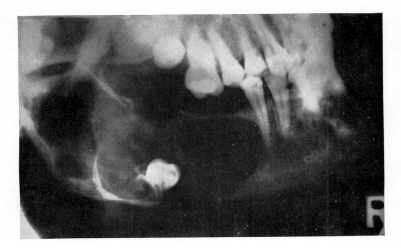

Fig. 11.2

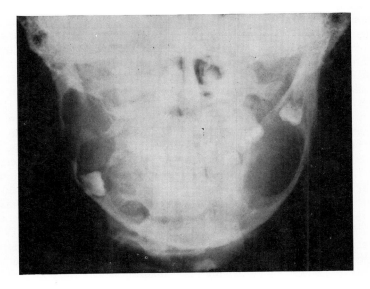

Fig. 11.3

Figs. 11.1 to 11.3 Lateral oblique and postero-anterior projections showing extensive bilateral mandibular dentigerous cysts in a girl aged 14. Bilateral dentigerous cysts were also present in the upper jaw.

patients with many carious teeth and roots, a surprising number of which will be associated with radicular cysts of varying size. In contrast, others are apparently 'immune' despite the presence in their mouths of several infected teeth.

Multiple primary dentigerous and radicular cysts may be treated by conventional techniques and recurrence need not be expected. Some cases of multiple and multilocular cysts from the older literature were almost certainly keratocysts, and some were unrecognized cases of the multiple jaw cyst–basal cell naevus syndrome.

Multiple jaw cyst syndrome

This interesting entity, often referred to as the multiple basal cell naevus syndrome, may implicate several structures or systems of the body. It consists essentially of multiple naevoid basal cell lesions, basal cell carcinomas, jaw cysts, skeletal anomalies and other soft tissue anomalies. Although Jarisch (1894) seems to have been the first to describe the disorder, Gorlin and his associates (1965) analysed 150 cases from the literature and catalogued all the known abnormalities. Indeed, the syndrome may be commoner than has hitherto been supposed, and is of special interest because of the high incidence of basal cell lesions of the skin and jaw cysts. Recognition of the disease may enable early detection and treatment of significant lesions and screening of asymptomatic relatives can be undertaken for signs of the condition.

The syndrome occurs equally in both sexes and has both a sporadic and familial incidence. When it occurs in more than one member of a family it appears to be inherited due to an autosomal dominant gene with high penetrance and variable expressivity. Yunis and Gorlin (1963) demonstrated a chromosomal abnormality. Cysts of the jaw were the presenting symptom in 50 per cent of Gorlin's series. They do not involve the primary dentition so that they appear from seven years onwards. The cysts are of the keratocyst type in the majority of instances but Rittersma (1972) records two cases in his series, one with a single layer of cuboidal epithelium lining the cyst and another with a mandibular cyst lined by ciliated and mucus-secreting epithelium. Not infrequently the cyst has an extrafollicular dentigerous relationship to an unerupted tooth. Sometimes a true (primary) dentigerous relationship is established (Payne 1972). Because there may be multiple cysts involving unerupted and developing teeth in a young subject, there may be a strong indication to attempt to preserve the teeth by employing marsupialization with the added risk of cyst recurrence.

A variety of skin lesions may be seen. Small, whitish spots or milia may be found, particularly around the eyes. The skin of the palms and soles of the feet is affected by a dyskeratosis which leads to the formation of characteristic pits (Mantoux's porokeratosis). Epidermal cysts may be found under the skin in most parts of the body, but are most often found on the hands. Basal cell naevi which vary in appearance from a whitish plaque to a raised excrescence, like a skin tag, may be found on the face, neck and trunk. Some on both exposed and unexposed surfaces may progress to an overt basal cell carcinoma. Basal cell skin lesions do not usually appear until the third or fourth decade. Most are less aggressive than ordinary rodent ulcers, but Rittersma (1972) reports a male patient aged 60 who died with multiple metastases from such a lesion.

The facies is often characteristic and includes the following physical anomalies: frontal and temporoparietal bossing of the skull, well-developed supraorbital ridges in males and ocular hyperteliorism. A number of papers refer to mild mandibular prognathism and three of our patients showed this feature.

A variety of other skeletal anomalies may be found in upwards of 75 per cent of affected persons. Bifid, fused and rudimentary ribs are among the more frequent phenomena. Occult spina bifida or fusion of vertebrae may be seen particularly in the cervical region. Bridging of the sella turcica, sternal deformities, Sprengel's deformity of the shoulder, shortening of metacarpals and bridging of the vertebral sulcus of the atlas are also recorded. Geminated and missing teeth and other dental defects are mentioned from time to time.

Other soft tissue anomalies are found occasionally, such as superficial fibromas, ovarian fibromas, lipomas and pigmented naevi. Block and Glendenning (1963) reported a failure of phosphorus diuresis in response to injections of parathormone (Ellsworth-Howard test), and Rittersma (1972) found calcium retention following a calcium load test in one subject. Lamellar calcification of the falx cerebri and in the tentorium and choroid is not uncommon. Murphy (1969) mentions subcutaneous calcinosis, and Rittersma (1972) has also seen this in the hands.

Agenesis of the corpus callosum and medulloblastoma may also form part of the syndrome (Herzberg and Wiskemann 1963).

A number of ocular anomalies including dystopia canthorum and congenital cataract (Rayne 1972) may be involved.

Treatment of the jaw cysts follows the lines laid down for the treatment of keratocysts in general. Proliferating strands of epithelium and daughter cysts are commonly found in the capsule so enucleation is the method of choice. Where it is desirable to attempt to retain a tooth involved in either an extrafollicular dentigerous cyst or a primary dentigerous cyst, the lining should be dissected away from the crown of the tooth. Sharp dissection with a scalpel may be needed. Unfortunately in these patients little of the root may be developed, so that the attachment of the tooth may be tenuous and its loss almost inevitable. In some cases the cyst may be marsupialized to permit further development of the tooth or to allow bone to regenerate over the roots of adjacent teeth. A further cyst may well arise subsequently at the same site, but enucleation can then be performed.

It is the nature of the condition that multiple cysts are produced so that both new cysts and recurrent cysts are likely to plague the patient until the late teens. However, further cysts may develop at any age, although with a much reduced frequency. Moreover, almost lifelong follow-up may be indicated to ensure that the patient is adequately monitored for the occurrence of basal cell skin lesions, so that unnecessary risks with these lesions can be avoided.

REFERENCES

Bennett, P. A. (1937) *J. Am. Dent. Ass.*, **57**, 591.
Block J. B. & Glendenning, W. E. (1963) *New England Journal of Medicine*, **268**, 1157.
Caldwell, J. B. & Thompson, A. C. (1955) *J. Oral Surg.*, **13**, 102.
Gorlin, J. R., Vickers, R. A., Keller, E. & Williamson, J. J. (1965) *Cancer*, **18**, 89.
Herzberg, J. J. & Wiskemann, A. (1963) *Dermatologica*, **126**, 106.
Ivy, R. H. (1939) *Ann. Surg.*, **109**, 114.
Jarisch, A. (1894) *Arch. Derm. Sypl.*, **28**, 163.
Maccaferri, G. (1953) *Archom. Chir. Oris Bologna*, 452.
McGregor, A. B. (1945) *Brit. dent. J.*, **84**, 35.
Murphy, K. J. (1969) *Clin. Radiol.*, **20**, 287.
Oliver, C. H. (1934) *Brit. dent. J.*, **57**, 591.
Payne, T. F. (1972) *Oral Surg.*, **33**, 538.
Rayne, T. F. (1972) *Brit. J. Oral Surg.*, **9**, 65.
Rittersma, J. (1972) *Het Basocellulaire Nevus Syndroom*, p. 140. Groningen: Niemeyer.
Seeman, G. F. (1937) *Int. J. Orthodont.*, **23**, 1138.
Sharland, R. J: (1948) *Brit. dent. J.*, **84**, 35.
Yunis, J. J. & Gorlin, R. J. (1963) *Chromosoma*, **14**, 146.

12. Miscellaneous Cysts

The calcifying odontogenic cyst

In 1962, Gorlin and others drew attention to an entity which they described as a calcifying odontogenic cyst, likening it to the calcifying epithelioma of Malherbe. Independently, Gold (1963) made similar observations and presented further cases. Gorlin, with others, published another paper in 1964 adding to the list of cases which they had found in the literature and giving details of new cases of their own. Many other examples have been reported since, all essentially similar to those originally reported.

There is no particular age or sex incidence, nor is there a preferred site in the jaws. Indeed, unlike most odontogenic cysts, some were found either in a saucer-shaped depression in the bone of the jaw or in the adjacent soft tissues. Indeed a cyst of similar appearance was found within the parotid salivary gland of a 7-year-old girl (Gorlin *et al.* 1964, Case 18). As has been indicated, there is a histological similarity in the way the epithelial cells undergo 'ghost cell' degeneration and calcification is also seen from time to time in craniopharyngiomas (Gorlin and Chaudhry 1959).

These cysts are lined by a stratified squamous epithelium in which the basal cells are differentiated from the rest by being taller and more darkly staining. Where the basal cells achieve a columnar shape the nuclei are found at the ends of the cells opposite to the basement membrane. That is, they undergo reversal of polarity reminiscent of the ameloblast. At intervals around the lining irregularly arranged masses of epithelial cells accumulate above the basal layer, and certain of these become strongly eosinophilic. At first, the outline of the cells and their nuclei can still be distinguished so that ghost cells are formed. Later, the outlines of the cells are lost and a hyaline mass is formed. Calcification may occur either before or after the outline of the cells has been lost. If pyknotic nuclei are incorporated in the calcified mass they may give it a superficial resemblance to cellular cementation or woven bone.

If the full thickness of epithelium is affected by the ghost-cell change the resultant mass may be shed into the cavity of the cyst. Epithelial downgrowths may be noted penetrating into the capsule at the periphery of the denuded area. In other places granulation tissue proliferates and penetrates the ghost cell mass. Giant cells appear in the granulation tissue and attempt to remove the degenerate epithelium.

Seward and Duckworth (1967) describe a thin, refractile lamella which may be formed over the connective tissue aspect of some ghost cell clumps. A collagenous hyaline material which stains similarly to predentine may be deposited against such ghost cell clumps and tubular dentine added later to the atubular material. Where such deposits of dentinoid and dentine are found in the capsule of the cyst, the presence of the refractile lamella on one surface may be evidence for the previous existence of a ghost cell mass at that site.

Gold (1963) describes a globular calcified material which he believes develops within the epithelial cells. Seward and Duckworth (1967) have noted similar single globules in thinner parts of the epithelium. Duckworth and Seward (1965) also noted concentrically laminated calcified bodies in the particular specimen described in their paper.

Several cases have been reported in which the lesions contained melanocytes – Lurie (1961), Gorlin *et al.* (1964), Duckworth and Seward (1965) and Abrams and Howells (1968). The latter paper is of particular interest because their melanin-containing specimen was from a Caucasian woman of 21. Mostly the pigmented variants have been from negroid subjects where the likelihood was that the pigmentation was racial rather than lesional.

Clinical features

Mostly the patient complains of a painless swelling, unless the cyst has become infected. The usual clearly circumscribed radiolucent image associated with a cyst is seen in radiographs. The bone cavities may be found in any region of the jaw. When they are small they are found between the roots of standing teeth. As they enlarge the roots of the adjacent teeth are either displaced or resorbed. Some cysts arise close to the periosteum and produce a saucer-shaped depression only in the bone. A radiolucency with a poorly defined periphery therefore results. Others are entirely within the soft tissues and produce no detectable change in the radiograph.

Because the lining contains calcified material, either calcified ghost cells or dentinoid, or both, small radio-opaque specks may be seen within the bone cavity and following the outline of the periphery. Such calcifications, too dense for their size for bone spicules, may be a clue to the diagnosis preoperatively. Only the adenoameloblastoma (ameloblastic adenomatoid tumour) produces a similar radiographic picture. In children the cyst may interfere with the eruption of adjacent developing teeth.

Treatment

Simple enucleation appears to be all that is necessary in most cases. However, Gorlin *et al.* (1962) record that in one of their cases (Case 12) the patient, a lady of 63, suffered a recurrence two years after enucleation of a solid lesion from the right third molar region. The recurrence was treated by jaw resection but there is no comment on the histological appearance of the periphery of the tumour. Duckworth and Seward's case (1965) had several unusual features. Apart from the fact that the lesion contained melanocytes, it was multilocular. Further, the larger cyst was encased in a thick layer of connective tissue and bone, the whole forming an invagination into the maxillary sinus. Numerous strands of lesional epithelium burrowed into the capsule and penetrated between the surrounding bony trabeculae. Small daughter cysts which also underwent the ghost-cell transformation could be found in the capsule of the major cyst, together with a variety of calcified dental tissues (other than enamel). As it happened the entire mass was removed from the cavity of the maxillary sinus. Should a similar lesion have occurred within the mandible, simple enucleation almost certainly would have left lesional tissue behind and a recurrence would have been likely.

The concept of dental lamina cysts

Remnants of the dental lamina appear to give rise to a number of cystic and related lesions, all of which form a keratinized or parakeratinized epithelium. These may be enumerated as follows:

Gingival and periodontal cysts
1. Epithelial gingival pearls of infancy (Bohn's nodules)
2. Gingival cysts
3. Odontogenic gingival epithelial hamartomas
4. Developmental periodontal cysts

Odontogenic keratocysts
1. Primordial cysts
2. Extrafollicular dentigerous cysts

Calcifying odontogenic cysts
1. Unilocular calcifying odontogenic cysts
2. Pigmented calcifying odontogenic cysts
3. Multilocular calcifying odontogenic cysts with affinities to odontogenic tumours

One of the justifications for including the calcifying odontogenic cyst in this group is the histochemical evidence that the ghost cells represent incomplete or abnormal keratinization and that some areas are fully keratinized (Gorlin *et al.* 1964, Komiga 1969). Indeed, Gold (1963) originally used the terms 'keratinizing' and 'calcifying odontogenic cyst' for this condition. Furthermore, like gingival cysts they may produce small cysts within the gingivae (e.g. Abrams and Howells 1968, case 2), or rather larger ones in the interdental bone like developmental periodontal cysts. In their occasional ability to produce burrowing strands of epithelium penetrating the capsule of the main cyst they can resemble the odontogenic keratocyst, although unlike the keratocyst frequent recurrence following surgery is not seen. The cuboidal and low columnar basal cells of the epithelium also resemble those seen in the keratocyst; even to the reversal of polarity.

Benign mucosal cysts

Terminology. Benign mucosal cysts occur within the lining of the maxillary sinus, arising mostly within the lining of the lower part of the affected sinus. Because their pathogenesis is uncertain, a variety of names have been applied to them, some descriptive and some reflecting ideas about their origin. They have been called non-secreting cysts, mesothelial cysts, retention cysts and mucosal cysts. According to Mattila and Westerholm (1968), Luschka discussed antral polyps and mucosal cysts (*Schleimhautzysten*) as long ago as the second half of the nineteenth century, and he considered they arose from mucous glands. Skillern (1923) viewed them as mucoid retention cysts arising when inflammation of the mucosa blocked the duct of a mucous gland, as did Hajek (1926). McGregor (1928) called them 'mesothelial cysts', believing that inflammatory exudate distended tissue spaces and the oedematous connective tissue between broke down, so forming the cyst. Mills (1954) believed that they arose in the wall of inflamed antra and suggested that the ducts of mucous glands became blocked, then distended and finally ruptured so that the secretions accumulated, stripping the antral mucosa from the wall of the sinus. He, therefore, conceived of a process similar to that which forms the mucous extravasation cysts of the oral cavity.

Hardy (1939) called these lesions 'cysts of the maxillary sinus', because he noted that they contained a thin yellow fluid rather than the thick gelatinous substance which is characteristic of a mucocele. Lindsay (1942) adopted the term 'non-secretory cyst' and Mills (1954) described the fluid as straw-coloured, sticky to the touch, sometimes containing cholesterol crystals and forming a gelatinous clot if left to stand. Eichelberger and Lindsay (1941) showed that the cyst fluid was similar to blood serum and also noted that it could coagulate. Wright (1946) described them as thin-walled, varying in size, containing a yellowish fluid and having thin blood vessels coursing over their walls. He pointed out that they are usually situated on the antral floor, have a wide attachment and rupture readily during removal; and that the inner wall has no lining epithelium. He likened them to a nasal polyp. Paparella (1963) adopted the term 'mucosal cyst', so avoiding the controversy over their pathogenesis, and Killey and Kay (1970) added the adjective 'benign' to emphasize their innocuous nature.

Most authorities seem to consider that they arise as a result of previous infection, but this seems at odds with the fact that the patients generally experience no symptoms and that the cyst walls and contents are free of inflammatory exudate. Indeed, only a few lymphocytes may be found in their walls. Dental surgeons will note some similarity between these cysts and solitary bone cysts, both as to their walls and as to their fluid.

Incidence

The benign mucosal cyst of the antrum is comparatively common and occurs in all age groups. As a result a number of workers have studied its incidence in routine radiographs. Millhon and Brown (1944) reported dome-shaped cysts in 24 of 600 consecutive radiographs. Ibsen (1944) examined 1760 maxillary sinus radiographs and found round shadows in 2 per cent. Wright (1946) reported 5 per cent in 1683 radiographs and Lilly *et al.* (1968) found an incidence of 2.7 per cent in panoramic radiographs of 1285 individuals.

Symptoms

Generally these cysts are asymptomatic, but occasionally vague and non-specific symptoms seem related to their presence and are relieved when the cyst is deflated or removed. Paparella (1963) describes a headache, frontal in nature and on the side of the lesion. Killey and Kay (1970) record a case which presented with a sense of fullness and numbness of the cheek. Mills (1959) mentions three patients who had a severe jarring pain while riding in a bus and Paparella mentions nocturnal facial pain. Some cysts may prolapse through the nasal ostium and subsequently rupture with a sudden gush of yellow fluid from the nose. Prior to rupture they cause nasal obstruction. Wright (1946) reported nine patients out of a series of 78 who had pain and tenderness in the face and teeth. In some cases infection of the sinus may supervene.

Signs

Generally there are no physical signs and the lesion is a chance finding in a radiograph. However, some may exhibit tenderness over the relevant cheek. Where the cyst has prolapsed through the nasal ostium a polypoid mass may be seen in the middle meatus and, if infection is superimposed, pus in the nasopharynx. These cysts vary in size from the minute to specimens which fill the maxillary sinus. Bret-Day (1960) and Killey and Kay (1970) have both reported cases which presented with symptomless buccal alveolar expansion, and Killey and Kay refer to another case in which the cyst prolapsed through an antro-oral fistula when the patient blew his nose violently. Transillumination curiously enough is normal, even when a large cyst is present.

Radiographic findings

The cyst appears as a rounded opacity within the maxillary sinus which differs from a dental cyst in that its outline is slightly flattened at the top and the periphery lacks the density which results from a covering of bone. It generally arises from the floor or lower lateral wall, and flops from side to side if films are taken with the head tilted. Lilly *et al.* (1968) noted that in no case was there evidence of related infected teeth or extraction sites. The cysts seem to enlarge very slowly, for films repeated at intervals may show little if any change in size. The rest of the antral mucosa is unthickened and apparently not inflamed.

Histopathology

The cyst is lined by a thin layer of oedematous connective tissue containing a few lymphocytes. Mills (1959) reports that cholesterol slits surrounded by giant cells may be present. On the sinus aspect there is a layer of normal respiratory epithelium and when these cysts have been reported as being lined by epithelium it is likely that the specimen was incorrectly orientated.

If a cyst is punctured either through the inferior meatus of the nose, or through the labial sulcus and the canine fossa, it may be aspirated. Often it will refill, but if it is possible to tear the cyst and rupture it into the antrum it will heal. Sometimes cysts disappear spontaneously, no doubt as a result of accidental rupture.

For large cysts which are causing symptoms the maxillary sinus may be explored through a sublabial antrostomy. The cyst usually ruptures but the bluish wall may be dissected away quite easily. An intranasal antrostomy is unnecessary and after haemostasis has been ensured the wound is closed.

Stafne's idiopathic bone cavity

Stafne's idiopathic bone cavities may be mistaken for cysts in the mandible. They are symptomless, and are discovered during routine radiography when they appear as round or oval-shaped radiolucent defects situated consistently beneath the mandibular canal and adjacent to the lower border of the jaw between the premolar region and the angle. Usually the recess lies in line with or behind the third molar (Fig. 12.1).

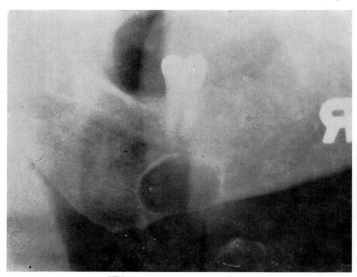

Fig. 12.1 A Stafne's idiopathic bone cavity can be seen in this lateral oblique view.

The area of rarefaction is well demarcated by a dense radio-opaque line. Sometimes the superior border of the lesion lies above the neurovascular canal. Below, it may perforate the inferior margin of the body of the mandible. It may be either a saucer-shaped depression or a deep concavity in the jaw; the dense bone surrounding it being a reflection inwards of the cortical bone so as to line the cavity. Sometimes the cavity is more complete with only a small opening on the lingual aspect. Stafne (1942, 1958) has recorded 113 radiolucent areas of this nature some of which were bilateral. Many were followed radiologically over a period of years and no change in size or structure was observed. The cavities varied from 1 to 3 cm in diameter. Stafne has expressed the view that the walls of the spaces examined were, in general, denser and thicker than those seen in bone cavities produced by epithelium-lined cysts of dental origin. According to the same author, no defects of this type have been observed in children. A suggestion has been made by him that such cavities might arise during development of the jaws by failure of the normal deposition of bone in an area formerly occupied by cartilage or by failure of subperiosteal apposition at the lower border. This theory was criticized by Rushton in 1946, who offered the alternative suggestion that the cavities might be the constricted remains of solitary bone cysts, adding the rider that 'until further information is available any interpretation must be speculative'. Rushton's assumption was considered acceptable by Thoma (1950) and Whinery (1955). In a discussion of Whinery's paper, Blum (1955) mentioned that some cases of latent or static bone cysts had been found to be eosinophilic granulomata. Jacobs (1955) explored two cavities, one of which was empty and the other filled by a part of the oral lobe of the submandibular gland; he believed that these were embryonic defects. Thoma (1955) reported operating upon such a case and finding a concave defect on the lingual aspect of the mandible which he attributed to erosion analogous to that caused by enlarged blood vessels in contact with bone. Two case reports were published by Fordyce in 1956. In one patient the outer cortical plate overlying the unilocular bone cavity was thin and lying in the defect was a mass which proved on section to be normal salivary gland tissue. By dissection it was demonstrated that this inclusion was continuous with the submandibular gland via a pedicle which extended through a perforation in the inner cortical plate. Similar findings at operation were noted in the second case. In commenting on the anomaly, Fordyce remarked that sialography should show in this type of case the extension of normal submandibular gland into the bony depression. From his own experience of such cases, it is MacLennan's (personal communication) opinion that the lingual plate is not perforated but displaced buccally. He suggests that this is the explanation for the failure of the cavities to fill in postoperatively unless surrounding cortical bone is removed. Richard and Ziskind (1957) described the investigation of a bony cavity in the lower left canine and premolar region. In the recess they found a solid mass of tissue which histologically resembled a

F

sublingual gland. There was a pedicle extension from the tissue which passed through a perforation in the lingual plate and traction on it caused movement of the floor of the mouth. The authors concluded that the pedicle was continuous with the sublingual gland. In a paper on the subject, Seward's (1960) view was that by virtue of constancy of position, uniform appearance, failure to change with time and occasional bilateral occurrence, the evidence was strongly in favour of these bone cavities being developmental in origin. He felt that the fact that they have never been observed in children did not exclude a developmental origin and quoted the more common developmental incisive canal cyst, which also has not been reported in the very young. Two lesions were investigated by Seward with sialography, and he demonstrated that the cavities contained salivary gland tissue continuous with the submandibular gland similar to those found at operation by Jacobs (1955) and Fordyce (1956).

Specimens of lymph node tissue have been identified after removal of the contents of defects by Bergenholtz and Persson (1963) and Thoma (1955). Simpson (1965) reports a mandibular defect which contained a pleomorphic adenoma and suggests that these lesions ought to be investigated first by sialography and then, if necessary, by surgery. In unrecorded cases explored by Kay in 1956 and Rowe in 1962 the cavities were found to be empty. All published reports have stated that the outer plate was thin and that perforations had occurred in the inner cortical plate.

From a survey of the literature it would seem that the cavities may or may not contain invaginations of gland tissue. A possible explanation for this fact is that if a developmental defect exists in the mandible and the submandibular gland happens to be superimposed over the cavity it is reasonable to expect the glandular tissue to extend into it. The authors agree with Seward (1960) who states: 'In view of the fact that the lesions are symptomless and non-progressive the exploration of further patients is hard to justify'. Apart from the diagnostic problem they present, these idiopathic cavities are of no particular importance, are non-pathogenic and require no treatment, though regular follow-up radiographs should be taken as a matter of interest and prudence. It should be stressed that the existence of a defect in the mandible does constitute a point of weakness especially if the lower border is involved and fracture of the mandible may occur at this site (Fig. 12.2).

In the course of an anthropological study of dry mandibles currently being undertaken by one of the authors (L. W. Kay), eleven idiopathic bone cavities have been encountered to date. All were situated either at the angle or below 678. The floor structure varied from rough and markedly corrugated to a smooth surface with minor irregularities and pitting. The edge of the compact bone depression was either punched out or shelving and the shape of the defect roughly circular or ovoid. Corresponding cavities in the region of the sublingual gland – above the

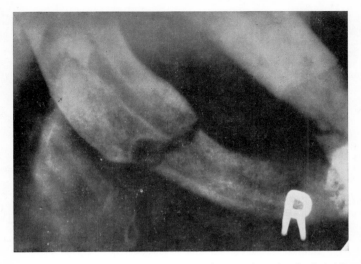

Fig. 12.2 This lateral oblique radiograph shows a fracture through a Stafne's idiopathic bone cavity. The fracture united satisfactorily following immobilization of the mandible with Gunning type splints secured by peralveolar and circumferential wires.

mylohyoid line – have been reported in the literature, but confirmation of their existence in anatomical specimens of the mandible is still lacking. The condition could, of course, represent an area of bone which has failed to ossify.

REFERENCES

Abrams, A. M. & Howells, F. V. (1968) *Oral Surg.*, **25**, 594.
Bergenholtz, A. & Persson, G. (1963) *Oral Surg.*, **16**, 703.
Blum, T. (1955) *Oral Surg.*, **8**, 917.
Bret-Day, R. C. (1960) *Brit. Dent. J.*, **109**, 268.
Duckworth, R. & Seward, G. R. (1965) *Oral Surg.*, **19**, 73.
Eichelberger, L. T. & Lindsay, J. R. (1941) *Proc. Soc. Exp. Biol.*, **48**, 191.
Fordyce, G. L. (1956) *Brit. dent. J.*, **101**, 40.
Gold, L. (1963) *Oral Surg.*, **16**, 1414.
Gorlin, R. J. & Chaudhry, A. P. (1959) *Oral Surg.*, **12**, 199.
Gorlin, R. J., Pindborg, J. J. Clausen, F. P. & Vickers, R. A. (1962) *Oral Surg.*, **15**, 1235.
Gorlin, R. J., Pindborg, J. J., Redman, R. S., Williamson, J. J. & Hansen, L. S. (1964) *Cancer*, **17**, 723.
Hajek, M. (1926) *Pathologie und Therapie der entzundlichen Erkrankurgen der Nebenkohlen der Nase.* Leipzig: Franz Denticke.
Hardy, G. (1939) *Ann. Otol.*, **48**, 649.
Ibsen, B. (1944) *Nord. Med.*, **27**, 1487.
Jacobs, M. H. (1955) *Oral Surg.*, **8**, 940.
Kay, L. W. (1974) *Int. J. Oral Surg.* **3** 363.
Killey, H. C. & Kay, L. W. (1970) *Int. Surg.*, **53**, 235.
Komiga, Y. (1969) *Oral Surg.*, **27**, 90.

Lilley, G. E., Butcher, G. L. & Steiner, M. (1968) *J. oral Med.*, **23**, 19.
Lindsay, J. R. (1942), *Laryngoscope*, **52**, 84.
Lurie, H. I. (1961) *Cancer*, **14**, 1090.
McGregor, V. C. (1928) *Otolaryngol.*, **8**, 505.
Mattila, K. & Westerholm, N. (1968) *Odontologisk Tidskrift*, **76**, 121.
Millhon, J. A. & Brown, H. A. (1944) *Am. J. Orthodont.*, **30**, 30.
Mills, C. P. (1959) *J. Laryngol. & Otol.*, **73** 324
Paparella, M. M. (1963) *Arch. Otolaryngol.*, **77**, 650.
Richard, E. L. & Ziskind, J. (1957) *Oral Surg.*, **10**, 1086.
Rushton, M. A. (1946) *Brit. dent. J.*, **81**, 37.
Seward, G. R. (1960) *Brit. dent. J.*, **108**, 321.
Seward, G. R. & Duckworth, R. (1967) *Dental Practit.*, **18**, 83.
Simpson, W. (1965) *J. Oral Surg.*, **23**, 553.
Skillern, R. H. (1923) *The Accessory Sinuses of the Nose*. Philadelphia: Lippencott.
Stafne, E. C. (1942) *J. Am. dent. Ass.*, **29**, 1969.
Stafne, E. C. (1958) *Oral Roentgenographic Diagnosis*. Philadelphia: Saunders.
Thoma, K. H. (1950) *Oral Pathology*, 3rd ed. London: Kimpton.
Thoma, K. H. (1955) *Oral Surg.*, **8**, 963.
Whinery, J. G. (1955) *Oral Surg.*, **8**, 903.
Wright, R. W. (1946) *Laryngoscope*, **56**, 455.

13. Differential Diagnosis of Cysts of the Jaws

Many bone-destroying lesions occur within the jaws and sometimes simulate quite closely the radiographic appearance produced by a cyst. Occasionally, too, certain structural anomalies and anatomical landmarks may also produce diagnostic confusion because of their radiolucent similarity to a cyst space. It is self-evident that clinicians must be aware of these entities and, in particular, the pathological variety, not merely in order to ensure accurate differentiation from benign cystic processes, but to avoid unnecessary speculation and, perhaps, serious delay in the recognition of malignancy. Such knowledge may even prevent an injudicious exploratory operation on, for example, an unsuspected cavernous haemangioma — a misadventure which could have serious or even lethal consequences.

Obviously, the first logical step to a good diagnosis instead of an inspired guess is a careful, factual account of the condition and a thorough clinical examination. With regard to the latter, the salient points have been discussed in the previous chapters. It is also important, when more than one jaw cyst is detected in an individual, to exclude a familial history and a genetic defect, for example, the multiple jaw cyst syndrome (Gorlin's syndrome, naevoid basal-cell carcinoma syndrome). Obviously a diagnostic decision may be influenced not only by the conventional sequence of clinical and radiological examination (including, if necessary, needle aspiration), but by biochemical investigations and, perhaps, biopsy.

There are several simple pointers to a firm, provisional diagnosis of cyst and these characteristics may also be helpful in identifying the actual cyst type.

Teeth
The presence of a discoloured dead tooth related to a periapical dark shadow, circumscribed in some cases by a white cortical line, supports a diagnosis of radicular cyst, whilst the absence of a tooth from the arch whose buried crown is seen, on radiography, to be associated with an enlarged follicular space can be indicative of dentigerous cyst. Occasionally, however, the associated tooth may be displaced into positions remote from the site of cystic origin, near the condylar or coronoid process, for instance, and lead to misinterpretation as suspected neoplasia. In contrast, whenever a radiolucent cavity is situated beyond the tooth-bearing area, for instance in the ramus, and provided that the

legitimate possibility of odontogenic keratocyst is excluded, then the extra-alveolar position must influence the diagnosis in favour of a non-cystic pathological process, such as a neoplasm, a metabolic disturbance or a fibro-osseous lesion.

A palatal swelling which lies behind vital central incisors and corresponds with a large radiolucent image at the site of the nasopalatine fossa will bias diagnosis in favour of a nasopalatine cyst.

Although its histogenesis is linked with an embryonal facial cleft, one can take the liberty of mentioning the nasolabial cyst, a soft tissue lesion, in the differentiation. This entity has certain striking characteristic features which assist in its recognition and exclude other pathological processes: it lies against the bone between the ala of the nose and the upper lip, obliterates the nasolabial fold, produces an external labial swelling and causes bowing backwards of the bracket-shaped line (as seen in periapical and standard occlusal radiographs). Stafne's idiopathic bone cavity (salivary inclusion) with its propensity for the posterior part of the mandible, including the angle, should present no difficulty. This defect is situated almost consistently beneath the mandibular canal and adjacent to the inferior margin of the jaw, demarcated by a reflection of the cortex, and it sometimes perforates the lower border.

Bony expansion

Invasive central tumours of the upper jaw present primarily as soft tissue swellings of the palate, as a result of early perforation of the bony shelf by invasion or simple pressure resorption. A malignant neoplasm which has produced such a swelling will also have produced gross destruction of the alveolar bone and this will be evident in radiographs. In contrast, a maxillary cyst usually expands upwards into the antral cavity, laterally and towards the nasal fossa; only at a late stage does it cause a palpable and visible bulge in the palate, and then it is probably associated with a lateral incisor and superimposed infection. Furthermore, a standard occlusal radiograph is useful for demonstrating that buccal expansion of the cyst may have modified the normal concavo-convex image of the anterolateral sinus wall so that it becomes a convexity. Swelling of both buccal and palatal tissues tends to occur only if the cyst has reached considerable dimensions, but with early buccal expansion alone the tooth of origin is probably the central incisor, canine or first premolar (Seward 1964).

In their growth, simple cysts in the adult mandible may attain a large size by longitudinal extension through the medullary bone, without any appreciable cortical expansion. There is, however, a tendency for cystic lesions anterior to the lower third molar to bulge outwards, affecting the outline of the buccal cortical plate rather than the lingual side of the mandible. This situation is in contrast to the behaviour of a neoplasm, e.g. an ameloblastoma, which as it increases in size, is prone to cause more obvious enlargement on both aspects of the jaw. Tumours may also 'expand' to a greater degree buccally and lingually − in proportion to the mesiodistal length of jaw involved − than do cysts. Whereas the mucous membrane overlying the latter remains normal in colour unless the cortical plate is breached, that covering a rapidly growing submucosal neoplasm is stretched and eventually the superficial blood vessels may appear more prominent than usual.

Aspiration

Comments on the value of this investigation have already been made in Chapter 4. Aspiration from radiolucent cystic or cyst-like lesions of the jaws, using a double wide-bore aspirating needle (Toller 1970), is a common diagnostic procedure. The rationale is well founded on the presumption that a cyst will be filled with straw-coloured fluid containing cholesterol crystals and that a keratocyst will have a keratin content. An apparently useful aid to the rapid preoperative diagnosis of keratocyst has been described by Kramer (1970). Keratinized squames can be demonstrated by the simple preparation of a stained H & E film of the cyst fluid, but the test has not yet been performed on a sufficiently large series to confirm how frequently it will provide conclusive evidence.

Solid tumour masses seldom yield any aspirated material, but some malignant lesions may undergo central liquefaction and the resultant 'fluid' can then be centrifuged and examined for neoplastic cells. When the clinician is unable to withdraw anything he will usually assume that he has entered a space filled with soft tissue. The presence of easily aspirated blood is suspicious of central haemangioma or aneurysmal bone cyst, and the aspirate will clot. However, it is also possible freely to aspirate blood from a cyst into which a brisk haemorrhage is occurring as a result of the needle puncture, or from a solid but vascular benign neoplasm such as an ossifying fibroma. Angiography may, therefore, be necessary to provide further information about the true identity of the abnormality.

The easy aspiration of air from a radiolucent area in the maxilla between the canine and the third molar implies that the antral cavity has been entered, and the diagnosis can be verified by injecting into the airspace about 10 ml to 20 ml (capacity of antral cavity is 15 ml) of sterile normal saline which will run out through the ostium into the nose.

If the cyst fluid is subjected to electrophoresis, it will be found that with typical apical, dentigerous or other non-keratinizing cysts there is a relative absence of large molecular proteins when compared with the patient's own serum, whereas albumin and globulin are present in normal amounts. On protein analysis, the total soluble proteins in these types of cyst are likely to be higher than 5.0 g/100 ml. In comparison, keratocysts are very low in soluble proteins, the level usually being under 4.0 g/100 ml (Toller 1970), and their fluids give characteristically pale electrophoretograms. Thus, this biochemical investigation not only has diagnostic value, but correlates fluid content with cyst behaviour.

Radiological features

In its classical form the cyst is shown radiologically as a rounded radiolucency with a sharply defined border marked out by a white line. As it grows the circular shape tends to be modified, and in the mandible, for instance, it may extend along the length of the bone, assuming a sausage-like contour. Needless to say, appearances can be deceptive and it is important to mention some fundamental radiographic patterns typical of some of the other pathological processes with which a cyst may be confused:

1. The presence of trabeculation and/or septa in an area of cavitation suggests the lesion is more likely to be a neoplasm, granulomatous or fibro-osseous disorder.

2. With rare exceptions, exemplified by the polycystic condition reported by Knight and Manley (1955), simple odontogenic cysts are not loculated. The 'partitions' which apparently enclose separate cyst cavities are actually ridges on the bony walls caused by differential bone resorption. Cortical perforation resulting in a dark patch on the cyst image may also give a fictitious impression of multilocularity. Nevertheless, diagnosticians may need reminding that a minority of keratocysts do exhibit authentic multilocularity.

3. A lobulated appearance with mosque-like indentations of the interdental bone between the roots of the standing teeth can be the insignia of the solitary (haemorrhagic, traumatic) bone cyst and is of diagnostic help when the lesion is discovered by chance radiography. The laminae durae of adjacent teeth are often intact and vital responses are elicited. With this condition, expansion of the normal contour of the jaw is uncommon. It is, however, possible to confuse it with disuse atrophy and the rare Gaucher's disease.

Special investigations

The biochemical laboratory may furnish corroborative evidence of the suspected nature of a lesion, for instance the specific abnormal proteins of multiple myeloma, or the raised plasma level of calcium and high urinary calcium (demonstrable by Sulkowich's test) in primary hyperparathyroidism. The final court of appeal may have to be biopsy.

Diagnostic interpretation

Awareness of the normal and abnormal is the best insurance against misdiagnosis.

Anatomical landmarks

Different projection angles may sometimes be necessary as well as very careful examination of the films, if errors of interpretation are to be avoided with normal variations such as a wide mental foramen or a sparsely trabeculated area of the jaws.

Periapical radiographs of the upper laterals may project the incisive fossa over the central incisor, thus simulating a periapical cyst. A misdiagnosis based on a hasty assumption can be averted by confirming that the apices are not denuded of lamina dura and that the teeth give positive vitality responses.

The shadow of an abnormally deep lingual fossa with a paucity or absence of bone trabeculae and outlined above by a prominent radio-opaque mylohyoid ridge may erroneously be labelled 'cyst'. An example of a normal bone marrow space, which may be open to misinterpretation as a lateral periodontal cyst, is the common triangular area of radiolucency deep to an unerupted, mesially tilted, lower third molar.

A well-demarcated dark area adjoining the lower incisors, which occurs when the labiolingual bone is very thin so that labial and lingual cortices are fused, can also closely mimic a cystic lesion in radiographic appearance and lead to a wrong diagnosis if the observer overlooks the existence of a normal nutrient canal pattern and the intact laminae of the related teeth (Stafne 1969).

The dark shadow of the concavity for the dentine papilla, which occupies the extreme apex of the developing root of a mandibular third molar, may be fortuitously superimposed upon the image of the mandibular canal. The resultant small area of uniform radiolucency can be very misleading and should not be confused with a small cyst.

Since a cyst in the upper jaw appears as a sharply edged, structureless radiolucency of circular or ovoid shape, its differentiation from the normal maxillary antrum – which it may occupy or overlap – should usually be clear-cut. The incidental existence, however, of very dark antral recesses, i.e. outpouchings from the main air space shadow in the alveolar, zygomatic, palatine and frontal processes of the maxilla may give rise to confusion.

The cardinal points of distinction between cyst and sinus are emphasized in Chapter 3 and a helpful criterion in the differentiation of a nasopalatine fossa from a non-odontogenic cyst of that name is carefully considered in Chapter 8.

Disorders of the maxillary antrum

The round, ovoid or dome-shaped mucosal cyst is probably the most common solitary lesion of the maxillary sinus, but in contrast to the odontogenic cyst it lacks a bony perimeter, whether it arises from the floor (the usual location), sides or roof of the antral cavity. Since it frequently undergoes spontaneous dehiscence or prolapses into the nasal passages, the mucosal cyst is unlikely to cause expansion or pressure atrophy of the antral walls; only two authenticated reports of buccal alveolar expansion have appeared (Bret-Day 1960, Killey and Kay 1970). Its degree of opacity is such that vascular grooves in the sinus wall can be seen superimposed on the greyish mass. The angle formed between the antral floor and the wall of an ovoid mucous cyst is obviously more acute than that produced by an odontogenic cyst 'invaginating' the floor of the sinus. A mucosal cyst does not generally exhibit intraoral signs or symptoms.

The antral polyp of an allergic or infective aetiology produces a grey shadow which can project from any of the walls of the antrum. If pedunculated the true identity of this mass of chronic oedematous, hypertrophied mucosa is more obvious, but it may have a broad base and more closely resemble a cyst. None the less, the distinctive characteristics of the lesion are such that it is apt to appear in groups and to be associated with mucosal thickening.

The rare occurrence of a polypoidal neoplasm, usually in cases of squamous-cell carcinoma, will present a thorny problem for the examining clinician. The radiographic appearance of any malignant neoplasm in the maxillary antrum may be merely that of a soft tissue mass without any special distinguishing characteristics. The earliest radiographic intimation that malignancy is present is bone destruction or loss of some portion of the floor or one of the walls of the sinus (Worth 1963). Identification of the lesion on such evidence implies that the case is at an advanced stage. The concurrence of signs and symptoms − a palatal or alveolar swelling accompanied by pain, denture displacement loosening and/or periodonticity of upper adjacent teeth − may aid recognition and ensure prompt differentiation from a benign cystic condition. Other sinister diagnostic features include involvement of the eye (diplopia, unilateral proptosis, optic atrophy), nose (epistaxis, nasal obstruction, epiphora), facial swelling and anaesthesia or paraesthesia.

Periapical conditions

A small, discrete periapical granuloma may resemble an apical periodontal cyst, but frequently the periphery of the lesion is less sharply demarcated than that of a cyst and it does not always extend as abruptly away from the surface of the root. Indeed, there is sometimes some fuzziness at the point where the lesion 'comes off' the apical lamina dura. While an encapsulated granuloma does not often exceed 1 cm in diameter, Oehlers' (1970) study of 412 periapical lesions is a pertinent reminder that periapical cysts under 5 mm in diameter do occur.

An early cementoma forms a connective tissue mass continuous with the periodontal membrane of a tooth, and this is represented radiographically by a well-circumscribed radiolucency in the periapical region. Some part of the lamina dura of the root may be lost if the lesion develops at the apex, but if the lesion is centred a little distance away from the root tip the lamina dura may persist intact. Multiple occurrence in the mandibular incisor region suggests this diagnosis, and the involved teeth will be of normal colour and vital. At a later stage there will, of course, be calcified spicules and eventually homogeneous masses of cementum.

Giant-cell lesions

The central giant-cell granuloma occurs more frequently in the mandible than in the maxilla with a site predilection for the posterior area. When noticed clinically as a bulging of the external or internal cortical plates, it is bluish in appearance, like a cyst, but firm in consistency. Radiologically, too, it may resemble the cyst and, to confuse matters further, be related to an unerupted tooth. Unilocular lesions may be oval or round with indefinite margins or sharply defined. Frequently, however, there are striations (internal trabeculation) across the dark area which give it a fuzzy appearance. Cavities, apparently multiloculated, are encountered, associated sometimes with resorbed adjacent teeth and the appearance of these is similar to that of keratocysts of the honeycomb pattern.

Fibrous dysplasia

Among the radiographic manifestations of fibrous dysplasia is the radiolucent pattern (Cooke 1957) due to fibrous tissue formation. This may have a cyst-like appearance bereft of a complete cortical rim, but if the bordering cortex is well defined it tends to be wider than that of a cyst and there should be some bony structure, i.e. faint trabeculae, within the substance of the cavity. If the lesion involves the teeth, the lamina dura may sometimes be lost.

Neoplasia and osteomyelitis

Most solid, slow-growing benign neoplasms tend to become rounded and compact initially, with a sharp margin. But in cases where teeth are pushed apart many such benign tumours are lobulated and have a partly crescentic outline. This is in contrast to the simple dental cyst, which will only tilt or move teeth very late in the adult jaw, after nearly all the supporting alveolar bone has been lost. Solid lesions also commonly cause resorption of tooth roots. Clinically a neoplasm which has penetrated the surface of the bone feels firm on palpation, not fluctuant like the cyst which has 'outgrown' the periosteum.

Central haemangiomas are usually discovered on routine radiography, the appearances being that of an atypical radiolucent area with a soap-bubble or trabeculated appearance. Adjacent medullary spaces and vascular canals are widened, so that the irregular outline has an indefinite border which blends into the normal architecture of the bone.

Although rare, it must not be forgotten that neoplastic processes, such as a solitary neurilemmoma, may involve the inferior dental or infraorbital nerve and cause a clearly defined, fusiform enlargement in the line of the canal. The position and possible disturbances of sensory function should help to clarify the diagnosis. If the bone of the jaws is involved, the lesion may be uniform or lobulated in shape, while extension may cause the overlying skin to be pigmented.

Cysts which appear circumscribed with cortical margins are usually sufficiently characteristic to exclude the diagnosis of malignant neoplasia or inflammatory bone disease (e.g. osteomyelitis), for the latter are often diffuse, poorly demarcated and, perhaps, perforating lesions. With established infective processes, a layer of subperiosteal new bone can be anticipated which is deposited alongside the jaw and can usually be confirmed by radiography.

Primary malignancies may either cause a complete loss of local bone leaving an irregular, ragged or feathery margin, or infiltrate widely with little obvious bone destruction. In the former case, teeth become loose and may appear to be 'floating in space'. Tooth resorption when it occurs leaves a spiky root. From the clinical viewpoint, central malignant new growths of the mandible cause expansion of the bone with pain, often accompanied by paraesthesia as a fairly early symptom. In the maxilla the invasive lesion may enlarge at the expense of the antral space before external evidence is apparent. A warning must also be given that osteogenic sarcomas are not invariably sclerosing lesions: they may be osteolytic and occasionaly so sharply defined as to masquerade as a benign condition.

Metastatic new growths in the jawbones are uncommon and are likely to be blood-borne. The rough, irregular rarefactive appearance of bone destruction from the direct extension of a primary carcinoma has already been mentioned. A solitary metastasis will also show as an ill-defined dark area, but it tends to originate centrally rather than at the alveolar margin and is usually in the third molar region of ramus of the mandible. Sometimes there are multifocal deposits. The primary sites for blood--borne metastases must be surveyed; although the bronchus, breast, thyroid and kidney are generally associated with osteolytic secondaries, the prostate may rarely be responsible. Lymphatic spread to the jaws occurs from a carcinoma of the lower lip to the mandible, and from the nasal cavity or sinuses to the maxilla. Clinically there may be overt signs of serious disease in the mouth, but the submandibular and upper deep cervical nodes may become enlarged from secondary invasion before the primary growth has produced intraoral changes.

Ameloblastoma. With regard to this neoplasm the radiographic appearances are variable, and confusion is most likely to arise when it is unilocular, for it can bear a close resemblance to a cyst. In whatever part of the lower jaw it grows, there is a tendency for both buccal and lingual aspects to be expanded. The posterior portion of the body of the mandible and ramus are the characteristic sites. With ameloblastomas of the cystic type, it is very unusual to find cholesterol crystals in the aspirated albuminous fluid. The intercystic partitions in the multilocular versions, which are composed of bone ridges and soft tissue, may either separate the lesion into numerous small cystic compartments (microcystic or honeycomb patterns) with marginal notching, or divide it into larger more variable loculi (soap-bubble pattern). With the honeycomb variety, in particular, there is considerable sclerosis of the adjacent bone. Even though some odontogenic keratocysts are divided into separate cyst spaces, which show individual variation in size, their locules are generally fewer than those of an ameloblastoma and their peripheral outline is sharp, not irregularly sclerosed. Clinically, a multilocular ameloblastoma may produce a knobbly enlargement, and there is a tendency for the transverse diameter to be greater in proportion to length than is the case with a simple cyst. Large examples of this odontogenic tumour produce a bulging pale pink mass with a granular surface which may break down forming a dusky-red ulcer. Paradoxically, erosion of tooth roots by an ameloblastoma is an uncommon sign radiologically, but not histologically. When revealed on a radiographic film, it takes the form of small, irregular erosions ('mice-like nibbles') at the edge or tip of the root. Although approximately one-third of large simple cysts cause truncation of adjacent tooth apices, since this is a benign pressure effect, the line of the resorbed root tip is frequently continuous with the smooth outline of the cyst. Often at the border of the ameloblastoma there is patchy or considerable sclerosis, and within the cavity a disordered arrangement of coarse trabeculae may be seen. When in doubt, biopsy material should furnish the diagnosis.

Adenoameloblastoma. An accurate diagnosis of this benign encapsulated lesion preoperatively is unlikely because it simulates a cyst too closely. In fact, although occasional solid ones have been described, the adenoameloblastoma usually has a central cavity. It is most likely to be confused with a dentigerous cyst. Suggestive, but not absolute criteria for diagnostic consideration are the site proclivity for the incisor-premolar region, the common association with an unerupted tooth, early appearance of the majority in the second decade, a clearly demarcated periphery and, sometimes, scattered calcific bodies within the radiolucency.

Fibromyxoma. A standard radiographic pattern cannot be ascribed to these lesions, but the radiolucent image of the single cavity with its scalloped outline may sometimes appear to be intersected by septa. The latter, however, are always straight and in complete contrast to the curved continuous wall of a cyst. The shape of the apparent spaces in a radiographic projection of the fibromyxoma are rectangular or triangular with the central portion traversed by fine, gracile trabeculations – the 'tennis-racquet' appearance (Sonesson 1950). Nevertheless, sometimes the structural details of the area are hazy and accompanied by coarse trabeculation (Killey and Kay 1964).

Fibroma (central, odontogenic and non-odontogenic; ameloblastic). The endosteal fibroma has sometimes the basic radiographic credentials of a cyst, i.e. uniform radiolucency and a smooth well-defined border. But apart from the great rarity of these conditions, this type of lesion may have a heavy lobulated outline and, in the case of the ameloblastic fibroma, be related to the crown of an unerupted and incompletely developed tooth. If clinically detectable, any of these lesions will be firm on palpation.

Miscellaneous diseases

Myelomatosis

The lesions of disseminated multiple myelomatosis are demonstrable radiographically as rounded, osteoporotic foci distributed throughout the skeleton, particularly the skull, sternum, spine, ribs and clavicles as well as the maxilla and mandible. In the jaws the porosity may be diffuse and accompanied by root resorption, loss of lamina dura and loosening of teeth. The clinical picture (recurrent back pain, progressive anaemia, weight loss, mental anaesthesia, tooth mobility) together with the radiographic changes and biochemical evidence (serum protein electrophoresis, Bence Jones proteose in the urine, sternal marrow puncture, etc.) contribute to a positive diagnosis.

Histiocytosis X

Both the chronic variety (Hand–Schüller–Christian disease) and the localized type (eosinophilic granuloma) can affect the jaws. With the former, multiple punched-out, osteolytic areas occur in the bones, but it may provide a diagnostic pitfall in the case of the mandible or maxilla if there are no concomitant oral signs such as swelling, ulceration of the gums and extrusion of teeth. Additional evidence of this chronic disseminated disease is likely to be apparent in the form of visceral lesions and the classical triad of skull defects, exophthalmos and diabetes insipidus. The eosinophilic granuloma is often single and appears more frequently in young children, particularly in the posterior region and angle of the mandible where it can simulate a dental cyst. Bone expansion accompanies the radiolucent defect and eventually the teeth are denuded of bony support and appear to be suspended in space. The true nature of the pathological process may only be discovered at operation and biopsy, but suspicious signs are marked mobility or spontaneous exfoliation of teeth, gross pocketing and failure of sockets to heal.

REFERENCES

Bret-Day, R. C. (1960) *Brit. dent. J.,* **109,** 268.
Killey, H. C. & Kay, L. W. (1964) *J. int. Coll. Surg.* **42,** No. 5, 504.
Killey, H. C. & Kay, L. W. (1970) *Int. Surg.,* **53,** 235.
Knight, J. S. & Manley, E. B. (1955) *Brit. dent. J.,* **99,** 419.
Kramer, I. R. (1970) Letter *Brit. Dent. J.,* **128,** 370.
Oehlers, F. A. C. (1970) *Brit. J. oral. Surg.,* **8,** 103.
Seward, G. R. (1964) *Brit. dent. J.,* **115,** 229.
Sonesson, A. (1950) *Acta Radiol.* Suppl. 81.
Stafne, E. C. (1969) *Oral Roentgenographic Diagnosis.* Philadelphia and London, Saunders.
Toller, P. A. (1970) *Brit. dent. J.,* **128,** 317.
Worth, H. M. (1963) *Principles and Practice of Oral Radiologic Interpretation.* Chicago: Year Book.

14. Complications

Fracture of the mandible

The presence of a cystic lesion in the mandible weakens the bone, and a fracture may occur as a result of comparatively trivial trauma (Fig. 14.1). The fracturing force may take the form of a blow on the jaw or a fall, but sometimes the mandible breaks as a result of the attempted extraction of a tooth related to the cyst, or even following tooth removal on the opposite side of the mouth. Occasionally, an undiagnosed cyst may become so large that fracture of the mandible occurs during normal mastication. If a cyst becomes infected and the underlying bone is involved, pathological fracture may be a sequel to bone necrosis It is rare for an infected cyst to undergo malignant changes, but when this takes place the untreated condition will inevitably progress to a pathological fracture.

Symptoms and signs

The basic symptoms and signs of a fracture through a cystic cavity are

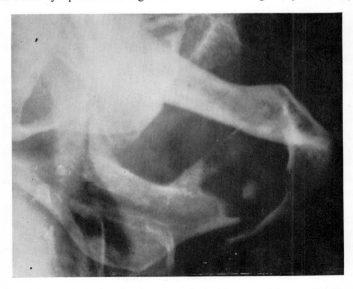

Fig. 14.1 Lateral oblique view showing a pathological fracture of the mandible through a residual periodontal cyst.

pain, interference with function, abnormal mobility, malocclusion, deformity, swelling, ecchymosis, crepitus and absence of transmitted movements. Additional to these features are the physical signs of the cyst itself which, of course, vary according to the position and dimensions of the lesion.

Treatment

The mode of treatment of a fracture through a cystic lesion depends upon the size of the cyst and whether it is infected or not. Modifications of treatment will also be necessary if a tooth is associated with the lesion when, for example, the fracture line runs through a periodontal or dentigerous cyst.

It is possible to enucleate a small mandibular cyst and yet leave sufficient bone on either side of the fracture line to ensure after reduction a wide area of contact between the ends of the fragments, which will lead to rapid healing of the splinted jaw. However, when the cyst is extremely large so much bone has been destroyed that little remains in apposition across the fracture line after the fragments are reduced, and therefore satisfactory resolution is unlikely to occur at the fracture site. Another important consideration is the nature of the benign cystic lesion. For instance, a fracture through a solitary bone cyst or a Stafne's bone cavity could be treated by immobilization without special concern for the cystic lesion, since in neither case does a true cyst lining exist. However, when a cyst sac is present and if, as in the case of a dentigerous cyst, there are one or more unerupted teeth in the fracture area, both lining and involved teeth must be removed to enable an uncomplicated bony union to take place.

With so many pertinent factors a cyst must be assessed on its individual merits. However, there are certain broad principles of treatment which should be taken into account and these can be discussed under the following headings.

1. *The nature of the cystic lesion.* The approach to the problem of a fracture occurring through a solitary bone cyst or a Stafne's bone cavity has already been mentioned. A cyst cavity which has no lining can be ignored, but in the case of all other types of benign cyst consideration may be given to the presence of the cyst membrane which is liable to become secondarily infected and so retard or prevent bony union. Ideally the cyst capsule should be enucleated before reduction and immobilization of the fragments. If the bone surrounding the cyst becomes infected and the fracture is complicated by bone necrosis, therapeutic measures must be introduced to cure this condition before hope can be entertained of successfully treating the fracture. The infected osseous tissue must be removed surgically and appropriate antibiotic therapy instituted. If there is gross bone loss, the gap in the structure of the mandible will have to be bridged by a bone graft after the infection has been eradicated.

When small residual defects are present in the mandible following the removal of diseased bone, a simple but effective treatment is to splint the mandible immediately accepting some displacement of the fragments.

If malignant changes have occurred in an infected cyst cavity the problem of treatment of a pathological fracture must be subservient to the therapy advised specifically for the neoplasm. If the malignant growth is treated surgically the resultant resection will have to be followed by bone grafting. However, this should not be contemplated until a sufficient interval has elapsed to encourage one to believe that recurrence is improbable.

If the tumour is successfully treated by radiotherapy an obliterative endarteritis may ensue in both the bone and soft tissue associated with the fracture. Probably this will preclude the possibility of spontaneous healing of the fracture, and may militate against the success of a bone graft.

2. *Degree of destruction of the mandible caused by the cyst.* It has been pointed out that if the enucleated cyst is small, there is an excellent prospect of accurate apposition of the fractured bone ends and uneventful normal healing following direct closure; whereas with a large cyst, failure of clinical union can be anticipated in view of the considerable junctional bone loss. Satisfactory repair and restoration of mandibular continuity in the latter circumstance will only be achieved if a bone graft is inserted into the defect after the removal of the cystic sac. If the cyst is not compounded into the mouth, this can be effected by enucleating the cyst from an external approach. As a replacement, either a block of cancellous with cortical bone can be used or chips of cancellous tissue can be inserted. The mandibular fragments are splinted by conventional means and if the patient is edentulous external pinning may be necessary. It is possible to insert a homogeneous bone graft by an intraoral operation and successful reports of the use of this technique have been made, but until wider experience is gained of its dependability, there should be a cautious approach to adoption of the method in this type of case.

An alternative surgical procedure for dealing with a pathological fracture through a large cyst cavity is to marsupialize the cyst, thereby removing the pressure stimulus causing osteoclastic activity, and immobilize after manipulating the fragments into a good position. In favourable cases bone deposition will occur beneath the fibrous capsule and the space will gradually decrease in size. The contour of the mandible at the fracture site will also remodel. To expedite the rate of bone regeneration within the cavity, a second operation can be performed to remove the lining of the marsupialized cyst after bony union has occurred.

Initially, after marsupialization the cavity is packed open with Whitehead's varnish on ribbon gauze and later a large gutta-percha bung is substituted. When the latter is inserted into the defect not only does it retain the patency of the fenestration, but it helps to stabilize the posterior fragment and so assist the fixation of the fracture. In an edentulous case after union of the fracture, an acrylic extension can be added to the patient's lower denture which acts as an obturator and maintains the opening to the cyst cavity.

In those cases in which sufficient bone remains in apposition to ensure union, the cyst lining can be enucleated and primary closure carried out. This is followed by an appropriate period of fixation using one of the standard methods of immobilization.

3. *The presence of infection.* If the pathological fracture occurs through an infected cyst, of primary importance is the control of possible contamination and, to recapitulate, it is essential to eliminate all evidence of infection before contemplating a bone graft procedure.

Carcinoma arising in an odontogenic cyst

Although rare in incidence, there is now well-authenticated evidence that apparently benign odontogenic cysts may undergo a malignant transformation. Recent cases of a primary carcinomatous change in the lining of periodontal, residual, odontogenic keratocysts and dentigerous cysts have been described by Hankey and Pedler (1957), Bradfield and Broadway (1958), Kay and Kramer (1962), Williams and Newman (1963), Ward and Cohen (1963), Hardman (1963) and Kramer and Scribner (1965).

In an excellent analysis of reported and unreported cases of malignant complication in odontogenic cysts, James (1965) refers to a survey conducted by Bramley, Erlich and Marsland at Plymouth and Birmingham which confirms the rarity of the condition — only one such case was discovered in 1166 patients investigated. In 1955 Bernier commented that he had not observed any malignant changes in the histological examination of 2000 odontogenic cysts.

Kay and Kramer have provided a résumé of the arguments and criteria by which malignancy can be presumed to have occurred in relationship to the wall of an odontogenic cyst. Possible alternative interpretations when an undoubted squamous cell carcinoma is associated with a cyst are as follows:

(1) that the initial lesion was an epithelial neoplasm, and the cyst cavity resulted from breakdown of part of the growth;

(2) that the jaw tumour was a metastatic deposit situated close to a simple odontogenic cyst with the primary growth located elsewhere in the body;

(3) that the carcinoma had arisen in a cystic ameloblastoma;

(4) that the cyst was not directly related to the malignant tumour, but both cyst and carcinoma arose in adjacent areas of the jaw and ultimately fused in some parts.

Following neoplastic transition, the behaviour of the growing carcinoma is usually that of a type with a low degree of malignancy. After inception, but before migration, the tumour will tend to grow into the cystic cavity so that the chances of cure are good if recognition and treatment are early. Lymph nodal metastases and dissemination by the bloodstream are often late events, although infiltration of surrounding bone and soft tissues may be well advanced. In one of Hardman's two cases, the patient died 13 months after the original biopsy, mainly from local extension of the growth. A pathway favourable to spread in the mandible is the mandibular canal, and if malignant cells gain access to the perineural lymphatics permeation along the neurovascular bundle could take place in either direction.

From his review of collected material, James noted a marked preponderance of affected males when compared with females (3:1), and a rise in incidence in the fifth decade with an age range from 23 to 79 years. In all, 37 cases were studied, but the sex was not stated in five of the persons concerned and the age was unknown in three others.

A bias was observed in computing the respective numerical indices of occurrence for the two jaws — cancerous change in a cyst happened almost twice as often in the mandible than in the maxilla. The study also affirmed that there was no special site for the initiation of neoplastic activity in a cyst lining. The general distribution of the cysts which developed a malignant character corresponded in location to positions occupied by uncomplicated cysts, and in the mandible the majority were situated in the molar region.

Clinical findings

Invariably the provisional diagnosis made after cases of this type are examined is that of an innocuous odontogenic cyst, and the underlying malignancy remains unsuspected until surgical exposure and biopsy. Often the cyst becomes secondarily infected and the lesion makes its first clinical appearance as a fluctuant swelling. In the edentulous patient the predominant symptom may be the poor fit of a previously comfortable denture. The unsolicited complaint of anaesthesia or paraesthesia may also invite suspicion of neoplastic activity, but such a presentation is not unusual when patients have large infected mandibular cysts uncomplicated by malignant disease. Expansion of the jaw, facial deformity, sinus formation, tooth displacement or pathological fracture are not exclusive to neoplasia in cysts — these signs too have been encountered in patients with benign cystic conditions. Findings which may have distinctive significance are extrusion of the cystic process through the covering mucosa followed by ulcer formation, failure of associated tooth sockets to heal, the loss in vitality and loosening of teeth in contact with the lesional tissue and severe or lightning pains.

Radiological examination

Despite critical study, radiographs may not reveal any changes which could be regarded as suggestive of neoplasia. The affected radiolucent area may have a smooth, sharp, corticated outline which is recognized as a typical appearance of an innocent jaw cyst, and even the loss of a cortical rim need only convey the possibility of a superimposed suppuration. The lack of a clear demarcation of the lesion from surrounding bone coupled with a sudden increase in its size detected on successive radiographs constitute presumptive evidence of a primary carcinoma. With infiltration of adjoining bone, the irregularity of the margins of the osseous defect together with frank exposure and gross displacement of the inferior dental canal could also be considered indicative of the presence of an osteolytic tumour mass.

A cyst-like cavity with peripheral notching raises the possibility of neoplasia, but the appearance is certainly not pathognomonic of that condition. Other radiographic characteristics which imply but are not conclusive of the existence of a superimposed malignancy are: (1) an extensive radiolucent area which has an ill-defined or ragged margin but no bordering layer of subperiosteal new bone; (2) implication of teeth with resorption of their apices or erosion of the sides of their roots leaving an irregular or spiky surface; (3) the loss of supporting alveolar bone so that the teeth in the osteoporotic area appear to be 'floating in air'.

Pathological examination

Macroscopic. The findings at operation may be: (1) the presence of a papilliferous mass invaginating the cyst space and infiltrating or adherent to the wall of the bony cavity; (2) uneven thickness or shagginess of the lining; (3) a nodular outer surface to the cyst sac; and (4) suspicious granulation tissue.

Microscopic. Sections of the material removed may show the conspicuous contrast of innocent epithelial lining in continuity with a mass of neoplastic tissue. There may be a hyperplastic type of cyst lining which contains cells exhibiting extreme pleomorphism, nuclear hyperchromatism and large numbers of scattered mitotic figures abnormal in form.

Treatment

The inferences deduced after reading the dental literature concerning malignant change in an odontogenic cyst are, firstly, that any pathological cyst-like condition should be removed without delay and, secondly, that there should be a careful microscopical examination with wide sampling and serial sectioning of the gross specimen.

The recommended method of treatment is a wide surgical resection, and in the lower lower jaw this will entail a hemimandibulectomy. Regional lymph nodes should be excised and submitted for biopsy. At a later date the continuity of the mandible could be restored by a bone-grafting procedure.

Obliteration of the maxillary sinus

When an expanding odontogenic cyst encroaches upon the maxillary sinus the antral bony floor becomes gradually attentuated. Eventually the cyst bulges into the air space and comes into contact with the lining mucoperiosteum. The adherence between cyst capsule and antral mucosa is maintained — unless infection supervenes — until the whole sinus cavity is occupied by the cystic lesion. Sometimes there may be little discernible distortion of the bony outline of the antrum, but expansion or erosion of the lateral and/or medial walls is not uncommon and even bone loss from all margins may be demonstrable. Treatment of the cyst is not only followed by restoration of the normal contour of the antral cavity, but it will be observed that alveolar bone re-forms around the roots of those involved teeth which were partially denuded of bony support.

Facial or cervical sinuses

External sinuses, either actively draining or chronic with a contracted, puckered orifice may result from suppuration within a cystic lesion of the jaws. Although a discharging sinus on the skin surface is usually near to the focus of infection, occasionally it may be located some distance away. After the cyst is treated the sinus opening will often disappear spontaneously, but an unsightly dimple may remain at the original site so that surgical correction is necessary. The problem of surgical excision may be complicated by an attachment of the depressed skin scar to underlying bone.

An elliptical incision is recommended to incorporate the whole area of scar tissue, and the incision lines are planned to coincide with the direction of the relaxed skin tension lines. The sinus track should be carefully dissected out using, if necessary, a silver probe or other instrument as a guide. After excision the surrounding skin is undermined so that the edges of the wound will approximate without tension. The subcutaneous tissues are then closed in layers using buried catgut sutures. It is essential to ensure that there is an interposition of soft tissue structures between dermis and the external surface of the jaw otherwise adherence of skin to bone will recur. The skin edges are accurately coapted and the wound closed with black silk sutures which are removed on the fifth postoperative day.

Nerve involvement with anaesthesia or paraesthesia

As the inferior dental nerve is displaced gradually by a growing odontogenic cyst, unilateral anaesthesia or paraesthesia of the lip is unusual. Unfortunately, however, the pressure of pus within a large mandibular cyst is sometimes liable to cause a temporary loss of impairment of labial sensation. Although the neurovascular bundle may lie immediately beneath cyst membrane, it is often possible to dissect the lining free from nerve tissue without postoperative sensory disturbance in the peripheral area of innervation.

When an alteration in labial sensation follows the temporary effect of pressure by abscess formation within the cyst sac the rate of recovery is rapid. A neurapraxia may ensue from operative trauma during the enucleation of a mandibular cyst, but full return of sensation to the affected mental region occurs within a short period and may even be present after two or three weeks. It is obvious that the more severe the degree of nerve injury the greater the delay in recovery, but regeneration always takes place after an axonotmesis so that normal sensory appreciation is restored to the anaesthetic area of the lip. Even in the unlikely event of a neurotmesis – absolute anatomical division – following a cyst operation, there will be considerable improvement in cutaneous sensibility during the subsequent 18 months. Probably this is due to the fact that the area of lip supplied by the inferior dental nerve has a collateral innervation from C2 and 3 and from the mental nerve on the opposite side.

After the removal of a large cyst in the maxilla it is unusual to encounter either altered sensation in the upper lip due to surgical interference with the superior labial nerves, or sensory impairment over the terminal distribution of the anterior superior dental nerves to the labial gingiva. Should either of these complications arise, however, recovery may progress irregularly but is invariably complete.

REFERENCES

Bernier, J. L. (1955) *The Management of Oral Disease.* St. Louis: Mosby.
Bradfield, W. J. D. & Broadway, E. S. (1958) *Brit. J. Surg.,* **45,** 657.
Hankey, G. T. & Pedler, J. A. (1957) *Proc. R. Soc. Med.,* **50,** 680.
Hardman, F. G. (1963) *Brit. J. oral Surg.,* **1,** 124.
James, P. L. (1965) Paper given at the Second International Conference in Oral Surgery. Copenhagen, Denmark.
Kay, L. W. & Kramer, I. R. H. (1962) *Oral Surg.,* **15,** 970.
Kramer, H. S. & Scribner, J. H. (1965) *Oral Surg.,* **19,** 555.
Ward, T. G. & Cohen, B. (1963) *Brit. J. oral Surg.,* **1,** 8.
Williams, I. E. & Newman, C. W. (1963) *Oral Surg.,* **16,** 1013.

Appendix

In order to evaluate the frequency and other aspects of clinical interest, 746 consecutive cyst cases seen at the Eastman Dental Hospital during an eleven-year period from 1 October 1959 to 30 September 1970 were analysed.

1. Relative incidence of individual cyst type

Table A.1 reveals the incidence of each variety of cyst. Taken collectively it will be seen that the periodontal group accounts for 67.82 per cent of the total number of cysts treated. In this category apical cysts outnumbered the combined figures for lateral and residual types by almost 2:1. Dentigerous cysts (17.4 per cent) were next in order of frequency, and odontogenic keratocysts were the least common of the odontogenic variety (3.3 per cent). Fissural cysts as a group accounted for 7.4 per cent of the grand total, and in the aggregate the numerical incidence for bone cysts was 3.88 per cent.

2. Age distribution at the time of diagnosis

The age distribution is annotated in Table A.2. The incidence of patients with cysts in the first decade was nil for all types with the exception of the dentigerous variety (16). The column for the second decade shows that this is an important age period for the occurrence of solitary bone cysts, and 37 apical cysts are recorded reflecting an upsurge in caries incidence. A rising trend in the number of periodontal cysts is noted in the following two decades reaching a peak in the fourth decade. The age periods between 21 and 60 years produce a consistently high level in occurrence of periodontal cysts, presumably because the liability to pulpal death from the relevant factors is greatest at this time. After 60 years of age — except for the residual cyst type — there is a marked fall in the number of cysts diagnosed and the incidence in the over-70 age group is negligible.

3. Sex incidence

There is a higher overall incidence of jaw cysts in males (481) than in females (265), which accords with the findings in Bradley's (1951) series. This probably reflects a tendency for females to be more dentally conscious than males. Table A.3 shows the respective numerical indices for each cyst type.

Table A.1 Incidence of individual cyst type

Cyst type	No. of Cases		Per Cent
Odontogenic			
Periodontal			
(*a*) Apical	360		
(*b*) Lateral	10	506	67.82
(*c*) Residual	136		
Dentigerous	130		17.4
Odontogenic keratocyst	25		3.3
Fissural			
Nasopalatine			
(*a*) Incisive canal cyst	41	42	[illegible] 49
(*b*) Cyst of the papilla palatine	1		
Globulomaxillary	13		1.74
Nasolabial	1		0.13
Median mandibular	0		0
Median fissural	0		0
Bone cysts			
Solitary bone cyst	23		3.08
Stafne's idiopathic cavity	3		0.4
Aneurysmal bone cyst	0		0
Multiple cysts	3		0.4
Total	746		

Table A.2 Age distribution

Type of cyst	No. of cases in age group							
	0–10	11–20	21–30	31–40	41–50	51–60	61–70	over 70
Apical	–	37	80	92	67	65	15	4
Residual	–	2	15	34	26	32	21	6
Lateral periodontal	–	–	4	3	1	2	–	–
Odontogenic keratocyst	–	4	3	2	2	7	6	1
Dentigerous	16	18	20	25	28	17	5	1
Nasopalatine	–	3	9	4	14	8	4	–
Globulomaxillary	–	4	6	3	–	–	–	–
Nasolabial	–	–	–	–	1	–	–	–
Solitary bone cyst	–	13	5	3	–	1	1	–
Stafne's bone cavity	–	–	1	–	–	1	1	–
Multiple	–	1	–	1	1	–	–	–

Table A.3 Sex incidence in individual cases

Type of cyst	Female	Male
Apical	139	221
Residual	46	90
Lateral periodontal	2	8
Odontogenic keratocyst	4	21
Dentigerous	40	90
Nasopalatine	13	29
Globulomaxillary	7	6
Nasolabial	–	1
Solitary bone cyst	13	10
Stafne's bone cavity	–	3
Multiple	1	2

Table A.4 Site distribution in individual cysts

Type of cyst	No. occurring in the maxilla	No. occurring in the mandible
Apical	277	83
Residual	84	52
Lateral periodontal	2	8
Odontogenic keratocyst	3	22
Dentigerous	49	81
Fissural	56	–
Stafne's defect	–	3
Solitary bone cyst	–	23
Multiple	1	2

4. Site distribution

The majority of cysts (all types) were situated in the upper jaw (472) and in comparison 274 occurred in the mandible, (Table A.4).

Of the 277 apical periodontal cysts positioned in the maxilla, the results showed that the greatest incidence was in the anterior region. Of those recorded in this area, approximately 60 per cent of the total number were associated with the lateral incisor. The explanation for the propensity of the second incisor to apical cyst formation is attributable to several causes and these are discussed elsewhere in the text.

Of the mandibular apical periodontal cysts almost 80 per cent arose posterior to the canine. All the solitary bone cysts were located in the mandible, and no fissural cysts (i.e. median mandibular type) were found in the lower jaw.

5. Mode of presentation

This enquiry (Table A.5) shows that 271 or 36.3 per cent were diagnosed by a fortuitous radiological finding and 199 (or 26.6) per cent as a result of secondary infection of a cystic lesion. Together radiology and infection accounted for 62.9 per cent of the cysts detected. The existence of a slow-growing swelling prompted 218 patients (29 per cent) to seek advice after a long period of procrastination. A minority of patients, 58 (7.9 per cent), were diagnosed for miscellaneous reasons which included pain without clinical evidence of infection, chronic sinus, interference with the fit of a denture, failure of teeth to erupt, discoloration of teeth and jaw fracture.

Table A.5 Mode of presentation all cysts

Type of Cyst	Radiological Finding	Superimposed Infection	Slow-growing Swelling	Others
Apical	128	107	98	27
Residual	34	43	52	7
Lateral Peridontal	1	7	2	—
Dentigerous	53	20	41	16
Odontogenic Keratocyst	5	7	8	5
Nasopalatine	18	13	10	2
Globulomaxillary	5	2	6	—
Nasolabial	—	—	1	—
Solitary Bone Cyst	23	—	—	—
Stafne's Bone Cavity	2	—	—	1
Multiple	3	—	—	—

Table A.6 Operative technique

Cyst type	Enucleation and primary closure	Enucleation and packing	Marsupialization
Apical	337	13	10
Residual	129	4	3
Lateral periodontal	9	1	–
Odontogenic keratocyst	18	7	–
Dentigerous	115	1	14
Nasopalatine	42	–	–
Globulomaxillary	13	–	–
Nasolabial	1	–	–
Multiple	3	–	–

6. Method of treatment

With the exception of the bone cysts, the remaining cystic lesions were treated either by enucleation together with primary closure or packing, and by marsupialization. In Table A.6 the respective figures for these operative techniques are reproduced. It can be seen that treatment by enucleation with primary closure accounted for almost 90 per cent of the patients. For obvious reasons the 23 solitary bone cysts and the three Stafne's bone cavities have not been included in the treatment statistics.

Index

Adenoameloblastoma, 159
Adrenaline 1:80 000, 52
Ameloblastoma, 158–9
Anaesthesia or paraesthesia of the lips
    associated with odontogenic cyst
    growth, 19–20, 167–8
Aneurysmal bone cysts, 132–4
    aetiology, 133
    pathology, 134
    radiology, 133
    treatment, 133
Appendix, 169–73
Aspiration biopsy, 31–32, 153

Benign mucosal cysts, 144–6
Bone cysts, 119–34
Bone grafting in association with enuclea-
    tion and primary closure, 58–9

Calcifying odontogenic cyst, 141–3
Carcinoma arising in an odontogenic cyst,
    164–6
Classifications, 1–8
Complications, 161–8
Cyst bung, 39
Cyst fluid, 31–32
Cyst of the papilla palatina, 113–14
Cyst pressure, 29
Cyst treatment in relationship to
    recurrence, 60–61

Decompression, opening into maxillary
    sinus or nose, 43–4
Dental lamina cysts, 143–4
Dentigerous cysts, 93–101
Diagnostic interpretation, 154–60
Differential diagnosis of cysts of the jaws,
    151–60

Egg-shell crackling, 18
Embryology of face in relationship to jaw
    cysts, 9–17
Enuleation
    and primary wound closure, 44–57
    and primary wound closure with bone
        grafting, 58–9

from the palatal aspect, 57–8
    secondary type and wound closure, 59
Eruption cysts, 75
Expansion of bone, 152–3
Extraoral radiography, 23

Facial or cervical sinuses, 167
Fibroma, central, odontogenic, non-odon-
    togenic, ameloblastic, 159
Fibromyxoma, 159
Fibrous dysplasia, 157
Fissural cysts, 14–17, 104–18
    possible origins, 14–17
Follow-up, 60
Fracture of the mandible in the presence of
    a cystic lesion, 161–4

Giant-cell lesions, 156–7
Gingival cysts, 93
Globulomaxillary cyst, 105–6
Gorlin's classification, 5
Gorlin's syndrome, 138–40

Histiocytosis X, 160

Incisive canal cyst, 107–13
Intraoral radiography, 22–3

Keratocysts, 62–74
    clinical features, 64–5
    contents, 66–8
    enlargement, 68–9
    histopathological features, 68
    radiological examination, 65–6
    recurrence, 69–73
    treatment, 73–4
Kruger's classification, 2

Lateral periodontal cysts, 89–92
Lateral radicular (periodontal) cyst, 89
Local analgesic solutions, 52
Lucas's classification, 4

Main's classification, 6
Maxillary sinus, obliteration of by an ex-
    panding odontogenic cyst, 166–7

Miscellaneous cysts, 141–50
Miscellaneous diseases, 160
Multiple cysts of the jaws, 136–40
Multiple jaw cyst syndrome, 138–40
Myelomatosis, 160

Nasolabial cyst, 114–17
   treatment, 117
Nasopalatine cyst, 106–13
Neoplasia and osteomyelitis, 157–8
Non-keratinizing cysts, 75–103

Odontogenic keratocysts, 62–74

Packing of cysts, 37
Periapical conditions, 156
Periapical films, 22
Periodontal cysts, 89–92
Physical signs, 18–21

Radicular cysts, 75–88
   enlargement factors, ·77
Radiographic interpretation, 24–9
Radiography
   extraoral, 23–4
   intraoral, 22–3

Radiological diagnostic techniques, 29–30
Radiology, 22–30
Residual cyst, 88–9
Robinson's classification, 1
Rotational tomography, 24

Seward's classification, 3–4
Signs and symptoms, 18–21
Solitary bone cyst, 119–32
Stafne's idiopathic bone cavity, 146–9
Stereoscopy, 24

Thoma-Robinson–Bernier classification, 2
Treatment, 33–61
   choice of operation, 34
   decompression, 43–4
   enucleation, 44–59
   follow-up, 60
   marsupialization, 35–43
   relationship to recurrence, 60–61
Treatment aims, 33

Vasoconstrictors, 52

WHO classification, 6–7
Whitehead's varnish composition, 37